HEALTH CARE ISSUES, COSTS AND ACCESS

VETERAN'S HEALTH CARE

ELEMENTS AND ANALYSES

HEALTH CARE ISSUES, COSTS AND ACCESS

Additional books in this series can be found on Nova's website under the Series tab.

Additional E-books in this series can be found on Nova's website under the E-book tab.

MILITARY AND VETERAN ISSUES

Additional books in this series can be found on Nova's website under the Series tab.

Additional E-books in this series can be found on Nova's website under the E-book tab.

HEALTH CARE ISSUES, COSTS AND ACCESS

VETERAN'S HEALTH CARE

ELEMENTS AND ANALYSES

CLAUDE DA COSTA
EDITOR

nova publishers
New York

Library of Congress Cataloging-in-Publication Data

ISBN: 978-1-62417-371-4

Published by Nova Science Publishers, Inc. † New York

CONTENTS

Preface		**vii**
Chapter 1	Health Care for Veterans: Answers to Frequently Asked Questions *Sidath Viranga Panangala and Erin Bagalman*	**1**
Chapter 2	"Who is a Veteran?" — Basic Eligibility for Veterans' Benefits *Christine Scott*	**31**
Chapter 3	Health Care for Dependents and Survivors of Veterans *Sidath Viranga Panangala*	**41**
Chapter 4	Veterans Health Care: Veterans Health Administration Processes for Responding to Reported Adverse Events *United States Government Accountability Office*	**51**
Chapter 5	VA Health Care: Weaknesses in Policies and Oversight Governing Medical Supplies and Equipment Pose Risks to Veterans' Safety *United States Government Accountability Office*	**63**
Chapter 6	Veterans' Medical Care: FY2013 Appropriations *Sidath Viranga Panangala*	**89**

Chapter 7 Veterans' Health Care Budget: Better Labeling of Services and More Detailed Information Could Improve the Congressional Budget Justification **123**
United States Government Accountability Office

Index **139**

PREFACE

The Veterans Health Administration (VHA), within the Department of Veterans Affairs (VA), operates the nation's largest integrated direct health care delivery system, provides care to more than 5.5 million unique veteran patients, and employs more than 258,000 full-time equivalent employees. While Medicare, Medicaid, and the Children's Health Insurance Program (CHIP) are also publicly funded programs, most health care services under these programs are delivered by private providers in private facilities. In contrast, the VA health care system could be categorized as a veteran-specific national health care system, in the sense that the federal government owns the medical facilities and employs the health care providers. This book provides an analysis of veterans health care with a focus on frequently asked questions; basic eligibility for veterans' benefits; health care for survivors and dependents of veterans; FY2013 appropriations; and weaknesses in policies and oversight governing medical supplies.

Chapter 1 - The Veterans Health Administration (VHA), within the Department of Veterans Affairs (VA), operates the nation's largest integrated health care delivery system, provides care to more than 5.5 million veteran patients, and employs more than 258,000 full-time equivalent employees.

Eligibility and Enrollment. Contrary to claims concerning promises of "free health care for life," not every veteran is automatically entitled to medical care from the VA. Eligibility for VA health care is based primarily on veteran status resulting from military service. Generally, veterans must also meet minimum service requirements; however, exceptions are made for veterans discharged due to service-connected disabilities, members of the Reserve and National Guard (under certain circumstances), and returning combat veterans. The VA categorizes veterans into eight Priority Groups, based on factors such as service-connected disabilities and income (among others). Dependents, caregivers, and survivors of certain veterans are eligible for the Civilian Health and Medical Program of the Department of Veterans Affairs (CHAMPVA), which reimburses non-VA providers or facilities for their medical care.

Medical Benefits. All enrolled veterans are offered a standard medical benefits package, which includes (but is not limited to) inpatient and outpatient medical services, pharmaceuticals, durable medical equipment, and prosthetic devices.

For female veterans, the VA provides gender-specific care, such as gynecological care, breast and reproductive oncology, infertility treatment, maternity care, and care for conditions related to military sexual trauma. Under current regulations, the VA is not authorized to provide, or cover the costs of, in vitro fertilization, abortion counseling, abortions, or medication to induce abortions.

Generally the VA provides audiology and eye care services (including preventive services and routine vision testing) for all enrolled veterans, but eyeglasses and hearing aids are provided only to veterans meeting certain criteria. Eligibility for VA dental care is limited and differs significantly from eligibility for medical care. For veterans with service-connected disabilities who meet certain criteria, the VA provides short- and long-term nursing care, respite, and end-of-life care.

Under certain circumstances, the VA may reimburse non-VA providers for health care services rendered to VA-enrolled veterans on a fee-for-service basis. Such Fee Basis Care may include outpatient care, inpatient care, emergency care, medical transportation, and dental services.

Costs to Veterans and Insurance Collections. While enrolled veterans do not pay premiums for VA care, some veterans are required to pay copayments for medical services and outpatient medications related to the treatment of nonservice-connected conditions. Copayment amounts vary by Priority Group and type of service (e.g., inpatient versus outpatient). The VA has the authority to bill most health care insurers for nonservice-connected care; any insurer's payment received by the VA is used to offset ''dollar for dollar'' a veteran's VA copayment responsibility. The VA is statutorily prohibited from receiving Medicare payments (with a narrow exception).

Chapter 2 - A broad range of benefits are offered to veterans of the U.S. Armed Forces and to certain members of their families by the U.S. Department of Veterans Affairs (VA). Among these benefits are various types of financial assistance, including monthly cash payments to disabled veterans, health care, education, and housing benefits. Basic criteria must be met to be eligible to receive any of the benefits administered by the VA.

For a former service member to receive certain VA benefits, the person must have active U.S. military service for a minimum period of time and meet nature of discharge requirements. Some members of the National Guard and reserve components have difficulty meeting the active duty and length of service requirements. However, a member of the National Guard or reserve components who is activated for federal military service and serves the full period of activation is considered a veteran for purposes of VA benefits.

The GI Bill Improvement Act of 1977 (P.L. 95-202) recognized the service of one group of civilians, the Women's Air Forces Service Pilots, as active service for benefits administered by the VA, and it also established that the Secretary of Defense could determine that service for the Armed Forces by a group of civilians, or contractors, be considered active service for benefits administered by the VA.

This report examines the basic eligibility criteria for VA administered veterans' benefits, including the issue of eligibility of members of the National Guard and reserve components.

Chapter 3 - The Civilian Health and Medical Program of the Department of Veterans Affairs (CHAMPVA) is primarily a fee-for-service program that provides reimbursement for most medical care for certain eligible dependents and survivors of veterans rated permanently and totally disabled from a service-connected condition. This report provides an overview of CHAMPVA and includes a series of questions and answers about the program.

Chapter 4 - The Department of Veterans Affairs' (VA) Veterans Health Administration (VHA) operates one of the largest health care delivery systems in the United States, providing care to more than 6 million veterans annually. Organized into 21 Veterans Integrated Service Networks, VHA's health care system includes 152 Veterans Affairs medical centers (VAMC) nationwide that offer a variety of outpatient, residential, and inpatient services. These health care services are delivered by physicians, dentists, and other providers and range from routine examinations to complex surgical procedures.

During the course of providing health care services, adverse events—clinical incidents that may pose the risk of injury to a patient as the result of a medical intervention or lack of an appropriate intervention, such as a missed or delayed diagnosis, rather than that patient's underlying medical condition—may occur, resulting in potential harm to veterans. They are required to be reported to appropriate VAMC staff through each facility's incident reporting system, or through other channels, such as anonymous phone calls or e-mails to VAMC staff, such as the patient safety manager or risk manager, according to officials. VHA policy requires that appropriate action be taken to evaluate reported adverse events. Once an adverse event has been evaluated, the VAMC may take actions that include correcting system or process issues and taking actions against individual clinicians when warranted. Specifically, actions taken against individual clinicians following adverse events may include adverse actions—ranging from admonishments to termination of employment; as well as actions taken to limit a clinician's clinical privileges, such as the reduction or revocation of privileges. Staff remediation activities, such as refresher training and proctoring, can be employed when adverse actions or limiting a clinician's privileges are not deemed necessary.

Recent adverse events have raised questions about the quality of care provided to veterans by VAMCs, and whether lessons learned at one VAMC are being translated into systemwide improvements. In response, members of Congress have raised questions as to the processes VHA has in place to respond to adverse events at VAMCs and take appropriate action, when needed, to address problems found within the VHA health care system. GAO was asked to describe how VHA responds to reported adverse events within its health care system. In this report, GAO describes VHA's processes for responding to reported adverse events within its health care system. In future work, GAO will examine the implementation of these processes at VAMCs. To describe VHA's processes for responding to reported adverse events, GAO reviewed and analyzed documentation that contains policy and guidance for these processes, including VA and VHA directives and handbooks. Specifically, GAO examined processes that enable VAMCs to determine the cause of an adverse event and assessed the characteristics of these processes. GAO also reviewed VHA's processes for taking action to help prevent an adverse event from recurring, such as correcting process or system deficiencies, using remediation approaches such as retraining and proctoring, and taking adverse actions against clinicians responsible for an adverse event. GAO also interviewed officials from VHA's Office of Quality, Safety, and Value, about issues related to quality, safety, and risk management and adverse actions. GAO's review was limited to VHA physicians and dentists, hereafter referred to as clinicians, as they are the primary types of licensed clinicians that practice independently at VAMCs. Furthermore, GAO's review was limited to describing VHA's processes for responding to adverse events, rather than all quality-of-care issues, such as those that did not rise to the level of an adverse event.

GAO conducted this performance audit from April 2012 through August 2012 in accordance with generally accepted government auditing standards. Those standards require that GAO plan and perform the audit to obtain sufficient, appropriate evidence to provide a reasonable basis for GAO's findings and conclusions based on GAO's audit objectives. GAO believes that the evidence obtained provides a reasonable basis for GAO's findings and conclusions based on GAO's audit objectives.

Chapter 5 - Department of Veterans Affairs (VA) clinicians use expendable medical supplies—disposable items that are generally used one time—and reusable medical equipment (RME), which is designed to be reused for multiple patients. VA has policies that VA medical centers (VAMC) must follow when purchasing such supplies and equipment, tracking these items at VAMCs, and reprocessing—that is, cleaning, disinfecting, and sterilizing—RME. GAO was asked to evaluate purchasing, tracking, and reprocessing requirements in VA policies and (2) VA's oversight of VAMCs' compliance with these requirements. GAO reviewed VA policies and selected two purchasing requirements, two tracking requirements, and two reprocessing requirements. At the six VAMCs GAO visited, GAO interviewed officials and reviewed documents to examine the adequacy of the selected requirements to help ensure veterans' safety. GAO also interviewed officials from VA headquarters and from six Veterans Integrated Service Networks (VISN), which oversee VAMCs, and obtained and reviewed documents regarding VA's oversight.

Chapter 6 - The Department of Veterans Affairs (VA) provides benefits to veterans who meet certain eligibility criteria. Benefits to veterans range from disability compensation and pensions to hospital and medical care. The VA provides these benefits through three major operating units: the Veterans Health Administration (VHA), the Veterans Benefits Administration (VBA), and the National Cemetery Administration (NCA).

This report focuses on the VHA. The VHA is primarily a direct service provider of primary care, specialized care, and related medical and social support services to veterans through the nation's largest integrated health care system. Veterans generally must enroll in the VA health care system to receive medical care. Eligibility for enrollment is based primarily on previous military service, disability, and income. VA provides free inpatient and outpatient medical care to veterans for service-connected conditions and to low-income veterans for nonservice-connected conditions. The President's budget request was submitted to Congress on February 13, 2012. The President's budget is requesting $135.6 billion in budget authority for the VA as a whole. This includes approximately $75 billion in mandatory funding and $61 billion in discretionary funding. For FY2013, the Administration requests $53.3 billion for VHA. This includes $41.5 billion for the medical services account, $5.7 billion for the medical support and compliance account, $5.4 billion for the medical facilities account, and nearly $583 million for the medical and prosthetic research account. The total request for VHA represents a 4.1% increase over the FY2012-enacted appropriations. Furthermore, as required by the Veterans Health Care Budget Reform and Transparency Act of 2009 (P.L. 111-81), the President's budget is requesting $54.2 billion in advance appropriations for the three medical care accounts (medical services, medical support and compliance, and medical facilities) for FY2014.

The Senate Appropriations Committee, Military Construction, Veterans Affairs Subcommittee approved its version of a draft Military Construction and Veterans Affairs and Related Agencies Appropriations bill for FY2013 (MILCON-VA Appropriations bill) on May 15, 2012; the full Senate Appropriations Committee reported the draft measure on May 22. The Senate Appropriations Committee-reported MILCON-VA Appropriations bill (S. 3215; S.Rept. 112-168) provides a total of $135.6 billion for VA and, within that amount, a total of $53.3 billion is for VHA for FY2013. The total amount for VHA is approximately $2.1 billion above the FY2012- enacted amount and $10 million less than the Administration's request.

On May 31, 2012, the House passed its version of the MILCON-VA Appropriations bill for FY2013. The MILCON-VA Appropriations bill for FY2013 (H.R. 5854; H.Rept. 112-491) provides a total of $135.4 billion for the VA and, within that amount, a total of $53.1 billion is for VHA for FY2013. The total amount for VHA is approximately $2.0 billion above the FY2012- enacted amount and 0.3% less than the Administration's budget request for FY2013. Furthermore, as required by the Veterans Health Care Budget Reform and Transparency Act of 2009 (P.L. 111- 81), the House-passed and Senate Appropriations Committee reported MILCON-VA Appropriations bills (H.R. 5854; S. 3215) provide $54.2 billion in advance appropriations for the three medical care accounts (medical services, medical support and compliance, and medical facilities) for FY2014.

Chapter 7 - The VA operates one of the largest health care delivery systems in the nation. Within VA, VHA provides a range of health care services for eligible veterans, such as primary care, inpatient and outpatient surgery, and nursing home care. In the past, VHA received medical care funds primarily through a single appropriations account. However, to "provide better oversight and receive a more accurate accounting of funds," in 2004, Congress established a new three appropriations account structure.

GAO was asked to (1) describe the relationship between VHA's appropriations account structure and VA's development of the budget request; and (2) examine how VA presents information about the three VHA appropriations accounts in its CBJ. To conduct this work GAO reviewed VA budget policy documents, VA's fiscal year 2009-2013 CBJs, prior GAO work on budget formulation at VA, and interviewed VHA budget officials.

In: Veteran's Health Care
Editor: Claude Da Costa

ISBN: 978-1-62417-371-4

Chapter 1

HEALTH CARE FOR VETERANS: ANSWERS TO FREQUENTLY ASKED QUESTIONS*

Sidath Viranga Panangala and Erin Bagalman

SUMMARY

The Veterans Health Administration (VHA), within the Department of Veterans Affairs (VA), operates the nation's largest integrated health care delivery system, provides care to more than 5.5 million veteran patients, and employs more than 258,000 full-time equivalent employees.

Eligibility and Enrollment. Contrary to claims concerning promises of "free health care for life," not every veteran is automatically entitled to medical care from the VA. Eligibility for VA health care is based primarily on veteran status resulting from military service. Generally, veterans must also meet minimum service requirements; however, exceptions are made for veterans discharged due to service-connected disabilities, members of the Reserve and National Guard (under certain circumstances), and returning combat veterans. The VA categorizes veterans into eight Priority Groups, based on factors such as service-connected disabilities and income (among others). Dependents, caregivers, and survivors of certain veterans are eligible for the Civilian Health and Medical Program of the Department of Veterans Affairs (CHAMPVA), which reimburses non-VA providers or facilities for their medical care.

---

* This is an edited, reformatted and augmented version of the Congressional Research Service Publication, CRS Report for Congress R42747, dated September 20, 2012.

Medical Benefits. All enrolled veterans are offered a standard medical benefits package, which includes (but is not limited to) inpatient and outpatient medical services, pharmaceuticals, durable medical equipment, and prosthetic devices.

For female veterans, the VA provides gender-specific care, such as gynecological care, breast and reproductive oncology, infertility treatment, maternity care, and care for conditions related to military sexual trauma. Under current regulations, the VA is not authorized to provide, or cover the costs of, in vitro fertilization, abortion counseling, abortions, or medication to induce abortions.

Generally the VA provides audiology and eye care services (including preventive services and routine vision testing) for all enrolled veterans, but eyeglasses and hearing aids are provided only to veterans meeting certain criteria. Eligibility for VA dental care is limited and differs significantly from eligibility for medical care. For veterans with service-connected disabilities who meet certain criteria, the VA provides short- and long-term nursing care, respite, and end-of-life care.

Under certain circumstances, the VA may reimburse non-VA providers for health care services rendered to VA-enrolled veterans on a fee-for-service basis. Such Fee Basis Care may include outpatient care, inpatient care, emergency care, medical transportation, and dental services.

Costs to Veterans and Insurance Collections. While enrolled veterans do not pay premiums for VA care, some veterans are required to pay copayments for medical services and outpatient medications related to the treatment of nonservice-connected conditions. Copayment amounts vary by Priority Group and type of service (e.g., inpatient versus outpatient). The VA has the authority to bill most health care insurers for nonservice-connected care; any insurer's payment received by the VA is used to offset ''dollar for dollar'' a veteran's VA copayment responsibility. The VA is statutorily prohibited from receiving Medicare payments (with a narrow exception).

INTRODUCTION

The Veterans Health Administration (VHA), within the Department of Veterans Affairs (VA), operates the nation's largest integrated direct health care delivery system, provides care to more than 5.5 million unique veteran patients,[1] and employs more than 258,000 full-time equivalent employees.[2] While Medicare, Medicaid, and the Children's Health Insurance Program (CHIP) are also publicly funded programs, most health care services under these programs are delivered by private providers in private facilities. In contrast, the VA health care system could be categorized as a veteran-specific national health care system, in the sense that the federal government owns the medical facilities and employs the health care providers.[3]

This report provides responses to frequently asked questions about health care provided to veterans through the VHA. It is intended to serve as a quick reference to provide easy access to information. Where applicable, it provides the legislative background pertaining to the question.

ENROLLMENT IN VA HEALTH CARE

Can All Veterans Enroll in VA Health Care?

Not every veteran is automatically eligible to enroll in VA health care, contrary to numerous claims made concerning "promises" to military personnel and veterans with regard to "free health care for life."[4]

Eligibility for enrollment in VA health care has evolved over time. Prior to eligibility reform in 1996, all veterans were technically eligible for some care; however, the actual provision of care was based on available resources.[5]

The Veterans' Health Care Eligibility Reform Act of 1996 (P.L. 104-262) established two eligibility categories and required VHA to manage the provision of hospital care and medical services through an enrollment system based on a system of priorities.[6] (See the **Appendix** for the criteria for the Priority Groups.) P.L. 104-262 authorized the VA to provide all needed hospital care and medical services to veterans with service-connected disabilities;[7] former prisoners of war; veterans exposed to toxic substances and environmental hazards such as Agent Orange; veterans whose attributable income and net worth are not greater than an established "means test"; and veterans of World War I. These veterans are generally known as "higher priority" or "core" veterans.[8] The other category of veterans are those with no service-connected disabilities and with attributable incomes above an established "means test."

P.L. 104-262 also authorized the VA to establish a patient enrollment system to manage access to VA health care. As stated in the report language accompanying P.L. 104-262,

> [t]he Act would direct the Secretary, in providing for the care of 'core' veterans, to establish and operate a system of annual patient enrollment and require that veterans be enrolled in a manner giving

> relative degrees of preference in accordance with specified priorities. At the same time, it would vest discretion in the Secretary to determine the manner in which such enrollment system would operate.[9]

Furthermore, P.L. 104-262 was clear in its intent that the provision of health care to veterans was dependent upon available resources. The committee report accompanying P.L. 104-262 states that the provision of hospital care and medical services would be provided to "the extent and in the amount provided in advance in appropriations Acts for these purposes. Such language is intended to clarify that these services would continue to depend upon discretionary appropriations."[10]

Which Veterans Can Enroll in VA Health Care?

Enrollment in VA health care is based primarily on veteran status (i.e., previous military service), service-connected disability,[11] *and income.*[12]

Generally, veteran status is established by (1) active duty service in the military, naval, or air service; (2) satisfying a minimum period of duty;[13] and (3) receiving an other than dishonorable discharge or release.[14] Exact requirements for enrollment eligibility depend on various criteria, such as when and in which component (i.e., active, Reserves, or National Guard) the veteran served. See below for questions and answers about returning combat veterans and members of the Reserves and National Guard.

Is Enrollment Different for Returning Combat Veterans?

Veterans returning from combat operations are eligible to enroll in VA health care for five years from the date of their most recent discharge without having to demonstrate a service-connected disability or satisfy an income requirement. Veterans who enroll under this extended enrollment authority continue to be enrolled even after the five-year eligibility period ends.

This special period of enrollment eligibility for VA health care was first established in 1998 and was expanded in 2007. In 1998, Congress, responding to the growing concerns of Persian Gulf War veterans' undiagnosed illnesses, passed the Veterans Programs Enhancement Act of 1998 (P.L. 105-368), entitling a veteran who served on active duty in a theater of combat operations during a period of war after the Persian Gulf War to be eligible to enroll in VA health care during a two-year period following the date of discharge.

In 2007, the National Defense Authorization Act (NDAA), FY2008 (P.L. 110-181) extended the period of enrollment eligibility for VA health care from two to five years for veterans who served in a theater of combat operations after November 11, 1998.[15] If returning veterans do not enroll during this five-year enrollment window (from the date of discharge), future applications for enrollment will be evaluated according to the Priority Group classifications described in the **Appendix**. For this reason, the VA encourages veterans to take advantage of the enhanced enrollment period.

Is Enrollment Different for Members of the Reserves?

When not activated to full-time federal service, members of the Reserve components have limited eligibility for VA health care services.

Similar to regular active duty servicemembers, members of the Reserve components may be eligible for enrollment for VA health care based on veteran status (i.e., previous military service), service-connected disability,[16] and income.

Reservists achieve veteran status and are exempt from the 24-month minimum duty requirement (as described above) if they (1) were called to active duty, (2) completed the term for which they were called, and (3) were granted an other-than-dishonorable discharge.

Members of the Reserve components may be granted service-connection for any injury they incurred or aggravated in the line of duty while attending inactive duty training assemblies, annual training, active duty for training, or while going directly to or returning directly from such duty. In addition, Reserve component servicemembers may be granted service-connection for a heart attack or stroke if such an event occurs during these same periods. The granting of service-connection makes them eligible to receive care from the VA for those conditions.

Is Enrollment Different for Members of the National Guard?

When not activated to full-time federal service, members of the National Guard have limited eligibility for VA health care services.

Similar to regular active duty servicemembers, members of the National Guard may be eligible for enrollment in VA health care based on veteran status (i.e., previous military service), service-connected disability,[17] and income.

National Guard members achieve veteran status and are exempt from the 24-month minimum duty requirement (as described above) if they (1) were called to active duty by federal executive order, (2) completed the term for which they were called, and (3) were granted an other than dishonorable discharge.

National Guard members are not granted service-connection for any injury, heart attack, or stroke that occurs while performing duty ordered by a governor for state emergencies or activities.[18]

How Do Veterans Enroll in VA Health Care?

To receive VA health care, most veterans must enroll by completing and submitting the VA's Application for Health Benefits (VA Form 10-10EZ).[19]

The following eight-step VA health care enrollment process is illustrated in **Figure 1**:

1. A veteran may apply for enrollment at any time of year by submitting the application for enrollment (online, in person, by mail, or by fax) to a VA healthcare facility. The application form includes information about the veteran's military service, demographics, and (as applicable) financial status.
2. Upon receipt of the enrollment application, the VA health care facility enters the information into the Veterans Health Information Systems and Technology Architecture (VistA) system, which creates an electronic record for the veteran.(If the enrollment application is submitted in person, a preliminary eligibility determination is typically provided at the time of application.)
3. The VistA system transmits the veteran's application information to the VA's centralized Eligibility and Enrollment System.
4. The VA's centralized Eligibility and Enrollment System establishes the veteran's record and queries the Veterans Benefits Administration (VBA) records.
5. The VBA returns information about the veteran's military status and/ or compensation and pension benefits.
6. The VA's centralized Eligibility and Enrollment System verifies the veteran's enrollment eligibility and shares these data with VistA. (If the enrollment system is unable to determine eligibility, it alerts the veteran's local VA medical center to take further action.)

7. When a determination has been made, the VA's centralized Eligibility and Enrollment System sends the veteran a letter with that information.
8. The veteran receives the letter from the VA.

The VA developed this enrollment process pursuant to the Veterans' Health Care Eligibility Reform Act of 1996 (P.L. 104-262), which required the establishment of a national enrollment system to manage the delivery of veterans' inpatient and outpatient medical care. Congress created the new eligibility standard to "ensure that medical judgment rather than legal criteria will determine when care will be provided and the level at which care will be furnished."[20] The VA classifies veterans into eight enrollment Priority Groups based on an array of factors, including (but not limited to) service-connected disabilities or exposures,[21] prisoner of war (POW) status, receipt of a Purple Heart or Medal of Honor, and income. (The criteria for each Priority Group are summarized in the **Appendix**.) Once a veteran is enrolled in the VA health care system, the veteran remains in the system and does not have to reapply for enrollment annually. However, those veterans who have been enrolled in Priority Group 5 based on income must submit a new VA Form 10-10EZ annually with updated financial information demonstrating inability to defray the expenses of necessary care.[22]

Are Veterans' Family Members Eligible for VA Health Care?

Veterans' family members are not eligible for enrollment in VA health care services. However, certain dependents and survivors may receive reimbursement from the VA for some medical expenses.

The Civilian Health and Medical Program of the Department of Veterans Affairs (CHAMPVA) pays for health care services to dependents and survivors of certain veterans. It is primarily a fee-for-service program that provides reimbursement for most medical care that is provided by non-VA providers or facilities. On May 5, 2010, President Barack Obama signed into law the Caregivers and Veterans Omnibus Health Services Act of 2010 (P.L. 111-163), which expanded the CHAMPVA program to include the primary family caregiver of an eligible veteran who has no other form of health insurance, including Medicare and Medicaid.[23] Health care services provided include counseling, training, and mental health services for the primary family caregiver. For more information, see *Health Care for Dependents and Survivors of Veterans*, by Sidath Viranga Panangala.

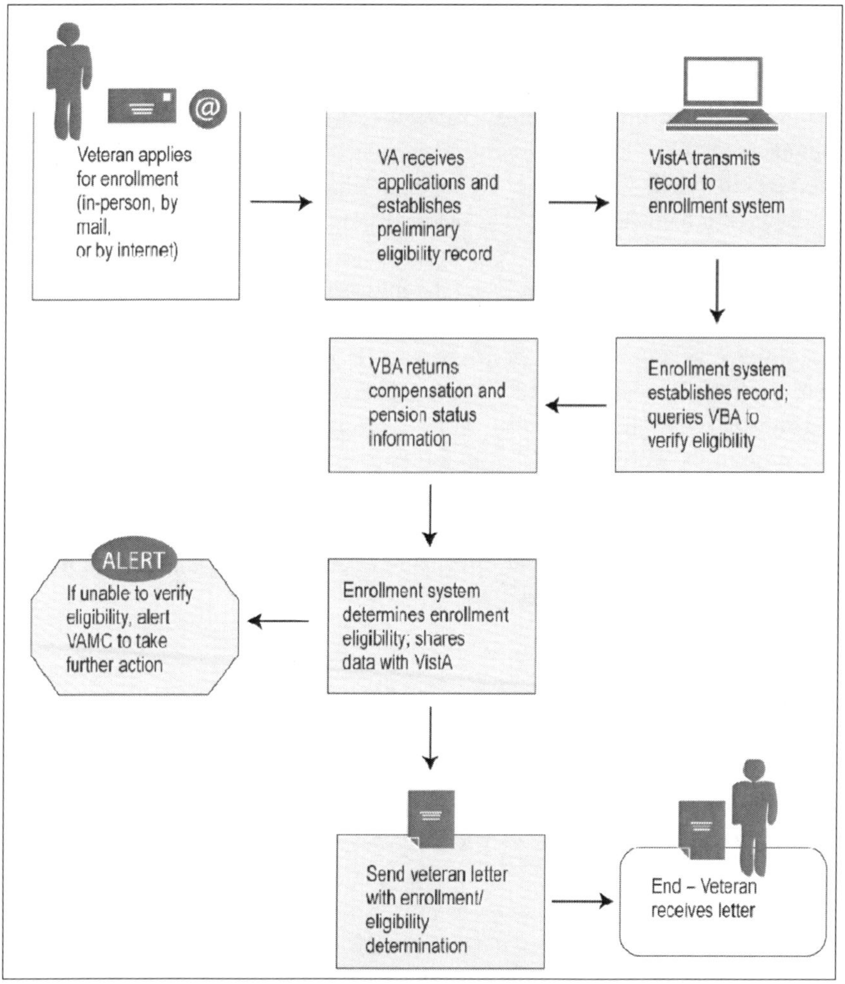

Source: Institute of Medicine, *Returning Home from Iraq and Afghanistan: Preliminary Assessment of Readjustment Needs of Veterans*, Service Members, and Their Families, 2010, p. 124, adapted by Congressional Research Service.

Notes: VistA = Veterans Health Information Systems and Technology Architecture; VBA = Veterans Benefits Administration; VAMC = VA Medical Center.

Figure 1. VA Health Care Enrollment Process.

MEDICAL BENEFITS

What Are the Standard Medical Benefits?

The VA offers all enrolled veterans a standard medical benefits package that includes (among other things) inpatient care, outpatient care, and prescription drugs.

The VA's standard medical benefits package includes a broad spectrum of inpatient, outpatient, and preventive medical services, such as the following:

- medical, surgical, and mental health care, including care for substance abuse;
- prescription drugs, including over-the-counter drugs, and medical and surgical supplies available under the VA national formulary system;
- durable medical equipment and prosthetic and orthotic devices, including hearing aids and eyeglasses (subject to limitations);[24]
- home health services, hospice care, palliative care, and institutional respite care;
- noninstitutional adult day health care and noninstitutional respite care; and
- periodic medical exams, among other services.[25]

The medical benefits package does not include the following:

- abortions and abortion counseling;
- in vitro fertilization;
- drugs, biologicals, and medical devices not approved by the Food and Drug Administration (FDA), unless the treating medical facility is conducting formal clinical trials under an Investigational Device Exemption (IDE) or an Investigational New Drug (IND) application, or the drugs, biologicals, or medical devices are prescribed under a compassionate use exemption;
- gender alterations;
- hospital and outpatient care for a veteran who is either a patient or inmate in an institution of another government agency if that agency has a duty to give such care or services; and
- membership in spas and health clubs.[26]

Does the VA Provide Gender-Specific Services for Women?

The VA's standard medical benefits package addresses the health care needs of enrolled female veterans by providing (directly or through access to non-VA providers) gynecological care, maternity care, infertility, breast and reproductive oncology, and care for conditions related to military sexual trauma (MST), among other services.

In addition, the Caregivers and Veterans Omnibus Health Services Act of 2010 (P.L. 111-163) authorized the VA to provide certain health care services to a newborn child of a female veteran receiving maternity care furnished by the VA. Health care for the newborn will be authorized for a maximum of seven days after the birth of the child if the veteran delivered the child in a VA facility or in another facility pursuant to a VA contract for maternity services.

Under current regulations, the VA is not authorized to provide or cover the cost of in vitro fertilization (IVF), abortions, abortion counseling, or medication to induce an abortion (e.g., mifepristone, also known as RU-486).[27]

Does the VA Provide Dental Care?

Eligibility for dental care is extremely limited, and differs significantly from eligibility requirements for medical care.

For VA dental care eligibility, enrolled veterans are categorized into classes, which form the basis for the scope of dental treatment provided. **Table 1** describes the eligibility criteria and scope of treatment for VA-provided dental care.

The Caregivers and Veterans Omnibus Health Services Act of 2010 (P.L. 111-163) authorized the VHA to conduct a three-year pilot program to assess the feasibility and advisability of providing private, premium-based dental insurance coverage to eligible veterans and certain survivors and dependents. Generally, survivors and dependents that would qualify for the program will be Civilian Health and Medical Program of the VA (CHAMPVA) beneficiaries. Under the three-year pilot program, the VHA would contract with qualified dental insurance carriers that will provide dental insurance and administer all aspects of the dental insurance plan. The VHA would administer the contract with the private insurer and verify eligibility of veterans, survivors, and dependents.[28]

Table 1. Eligibility Criteria and Scope of Treatment for VA Dental Care

Classification	Eligibility Criteria	Scope of Treatment Provided
Class I	Veteran has a service-connected compensable (disability compensation paid) dental condition	Any necessary dental treatment to maintain or restore oral health and masticatory function, including repeat care
Class II	Veteran has a service-connected noncompensable dental condition (not subject to disability compensation) shown to have been in existence at the time of discharge or release from active duty service, which took place after September 30, 1981, if: The veteran served at least 180 days (or 90 days if a veteran of the Gulf War era), and The veteran's DD214[a] does not bear certification that the veteran was provided, within 90 days immediately prior to discharge or release, a complete dental examination (including dental x-rays) and all appropriate dental treatment indicated by the examination to be needed, and Application for treatment is received within 180 days of discharge	A one-time course of dental treatment of the service-connected noncompensable dental condition
Class II (a)	Veteran has a service-connected noncompensable dental condition or disability determined as resulting from combat wounds or service trauma	Any necessary dental treatment for the correction of the service-connected condition. Generally, a Dental Trauma Rating or VA Regional Office Rating Decision letter identifies the tooth/teeth eligible for care.
Class II(b)	Veteran is homeless or are otherwise enrolled in certain VA-sponsored rehabilitation programs	A one-time course of dental treatment
Class II(c)	Veteran is a former prisoner of war (POW)	Any necessary dental treatment to maintain or restore oral health and masticatory function, including repeat care
Class III	Veteran has a nonservice-connected dental disability professionally determined to be aggravating a service-connected medical condition	A one-time course of dental treatment to treat only the oral condition that is directly impacting the management of the service-connected medical condition. Eligibility for each new course of dental treatment is a based on a new dental evaluation.
Class IV	Veteran whose service-connected disabilities have been rated at 100% or who is receiving the 100% rating by reason of individual unemployability.	Any necessary dental treatment to maintain or restore oral health and masticatory function, including repeat care

Table 1. (Continued)

Classification	Eligibility Criteria	Scope of Treatment Provided
Class V	Veteran who is approved for VA vocational rehabilitation training and who requires dental treatment to participate in the training	Dental care to the extent needed to meet any of the following goals: 1. make possible his or her entrance into a rehabilitation program; 2. achieve the goals of the veteran's vocational rehabilitation program; 3. prevent interruption of a rehabilitation program; 4. hasten the return to a rehabilitation program of a veteran in interrupted or leave status; 5. hasten the return to a rehabilitation program of a veteran placed in discontinued status because of a dental condition; 6. secure and adjust to employment during the period of employment assistance; or 7. enable the veteran to achieve maximum independence in daily living
Class VI	Veteran scheduled for admission to VA medical center or otherwise receiving care and services, if dental care is reasonably necessary to the provision of such care and services, that is, a dental condition is complicating a medical condition currently under treatment. (Examples: patients scheduled for cardiac surgery, knee, hip, joint replacement surgery, or organ transplant surgery may receive pre-bed care to eliminate dental infection prior to their surgery to help insure successful medical treatment)	A one-time course of dental treatment to treat conditions that directly impact the management of the nonservice-connected medical condition

Source: 38 C.F.R. §§ 17.160-162 and Department of Veterans Affairs, Veterans Health Administration, *Criteria and Standards for Dental Program*, VHA Handbook 1130.01, December 25, 2008.

a. When servicemembers separate from active military service, they each receive a certificate of release or discharge from active duty, known as a DD-214. The DD-214 provides the member and the service with a concise record of a period of service with the Armed Forces at the time of the member's separation, discharge, or change in military status (reserve/active duty). In addition, the form serves as an authoritative source of information for both governmental agencies and the Armed Forces for purposes of employment, benefit, and reenlistment eligibility, respectively.

Does the VA Provide Hearing Aids and Eyeglasses?

Generally, the VA provides audiology and eye care services (including preventive care services and routine vision testing) for all enrolled veterans. The VA does not provide hearing aids or eye glasses for normally occurring hearing or vision loss.

Hearing aids and eyeglasses are provided to the following veterans:[29]

- Veterans with any compensable service-connected disability.
- Veterans who are former prisoners of war (POWs).
- Veterans who were awarded a Purple Heart.
- Veterans receiving compensation for an injury, or an aggravation of an injury, that occurred as the result of VA treatment.
- Veterans in receipt of an increased pension based on being permanently housebound and in need of regular aid and attendance.
- Veterans with hearing or vision impairment resulting from diseases or the existence of another medical condition for which the veteran is receiving care or services from VA, or which resulted from treatment of that medical condition (e.g., stroke, polytrauma, traumatic brain injury, diabetes, multiple sclerosis, vascular disease, geriatric chronic illnesses, toxicity from drugs, ocular photosensitivity from drugs, cataract surgery, and/or other surgeries performed on the eye, ear, or brain resulting in a vision or hearing impairment).
- Veterans with significant functional or cognitive impairment evidenced by deficiencies in the ability to perform activities of daily living.[30]
- Veterans who have hearing and/or vision impairment severe enough that it interferes with their ability to participate actively in their own medical treatment and to reduce the impact of dual sensory impairment (combined hearing and vision loss).

Does the VA Provide Long-Term Care?

The VA provides long-term care services (including residential, home-based, and community-based care) for veterans meeting specified criteria, which may include service-connected conditions and the need for such care.

The Veterans Millennium Healthcare and Benefits Act (P.L. 106-117) requires the VA to provide nursing home services to all enrolled veterans who are 70% or more service-connected disabled, or 60% or more service-connected disabled and unemployable and in need of such care, or who are service-connected for a condition that makes such care necessary.[31]

The VA meets the requirements of P.L. 106-117 by providing short-and long-term nursing care, respite, and end-of-life care through three different settings: Community Living Centers (CLCs) located on VA medical campuses; contracted care in Community Nursing Homes (CNH); and through the State Veterans Nursing Home (SVNH) program.

Under the SVNH program, the VA subsidizes state-operated, long-term care facilities for veterans through a grant and per diem program in states that have petitioned the VA to build and operate a SVNH. The SVNH program primarily provides long-stay, maintenance-level care.

Each SVNH is owned and operated by its host state; however, approximately two-thirds of new construction costs and about one-third of per diem costs are provided by the VA. For those veterans who are 70% or more service-connected disabled and reside in a SVNH, the VA provides the full cost of care.

The VA provides a range of non-institutional home and community based services for veterans, which include the following:

- Skilled Home Care—the Purchased Skilled Home Care Program (formerly known as fee basis home care) is a professional home care service that is purchased from private-sector providers by every VA medical center. A VA primary care provider must recommend Skilled Home Care in order for a veteran to receive it. The professional home care services program covers mostly nursing services, including medical care, social services, occupational therapy, physical therapy, skilled nursing care, and speech and language pathology.
- Home Based Primary Care—This program (formerly known as Hospital Based Home Care) began in 1970 and provides medical care to chronically ill or disabled veterans in their own homes through an interdisciplinary treatment team. These services are paid for by the VA and provided by VA personnel.
- Veteran-Directed Home & Community Based Care—The VA partners with federal Area Agencies on Aging to purchase needed services. This program allows the veteran to decide on a case mix of services to best meet care needs and those of the caregiver.
- Spinal Cord Injury/Disorders Bowel & Bladder Care—These programs provide specialized home care services for veterans with

spinal cord injuries and related disorders. Services include respite care, long-term care, bowel and bladder care, and caregiver education to veterans.

- Homemaker/Home Health Aide—This program began in 1993 and provides assistance with personal care and related support services for veterans in their own homes through the homemaker/home health aide (H/HHA) benefit. H/HHA services may include assistance with activities of daily living (ADLs), as well as instrumental activities of daily living (IADLs).[32] Eligibility for the H/HHA program is based on a clinical judgment by the H/HHA Coordinator and interdisciplinary team that determines if the veteran would, in the absence of H/HHA services, require nursing home equivalent care. The VA pays for these services. H/HHA services are provided by contracted providers. H/HHAs are personnel who are trained and have completed a competency evaluation, and are placed under the general supervision of a nurse.
- Community Residential Care (CRC)[33]—CRC is a form of enriched housing that provides health care supervision to eligible veterans not in need of hospital or nursing home care, but who, because of medical and psychiatric and/or psychosocial limitations, as determined through a statement of needed care, are not able to live independently and have no suitable family or significant others to provide the needed supervision and supportive care. CRCs currently encompass
    - assisted living facilities;
    - personal care homes;
    - family care homes;
    - psychiatric community residential care homes; and
    - medical foster homes.

In general, each of the settings listed above must provide room, board, assistance with Activities of Daily Living (ADL), and supervision as determined on an individual basis.

The individual veteran makes the final choice of facility, and the cost of residential care is financed by the veteran's own resources. However, placement in residential settings is subject to inspection and approval by the appropriate VA medical center.

Does the VA Pay for Medical Care at Non-VA Facilities?

Under certain circumstances, the VA may reimburse non-VA providers for health care services rendered to VA-enrolled veterans on a fee-for-service basis.

Current law authorizes the VA to use Fee Basis Care under the following circumstances: (1) when a clinical service cannot be provided at a VA medical center (VAMC); (2) when a veteran is unable to access VA health care facilities due to geographic inaccessibility; or (3) in emergencies when delays could lead to life-threatening situations.[34] Fee Basis Care may include outpatient care, inpatient care, emergency care, medical transportation, and dental services.[35]

Does the VA Pay for Emergency Care at Non-VA Facilities?

The VA may pay for emergency care provided to enrolled veterans by non-VA providers based on several factors, such as whether the care is for a service-connected condition.

Generally, to be eligible for non-VA emergency care reimbursement veterans must

- be enrolled in the VA health care system, and
- have received VA medical services within the 24-month period preceding the furnishing of emergency treatment.[36]

Once these general eligibility criteria are met, emergency care reimbursement falls into two categories: (1) payment or reimbursement of emergency care for veterans for a service-connected disability[37] and (2) payment or reimbursement of emergency care for veterans for a nonservice-connected disability.[38] The distinct eligibility criteria for each of the two categories are summarized in **Table 2**.

Costs to Veterans and Insurance Collections

Do Veterans Have to Pay for Their Care?

Whether a veteran is required to pay for VA health care services depends primarily on (1) whether the condition being treated is service-connected, and/or (2) the veteran's enrollment Priority Group.[39]

Veterans who are enrolled in the VA health care system do not pay any premiums; however, some veterans are required to pay copayments for medical services and outpatient medications related to the treatment of a nonservice-connected condition. **Table 3** summarizes which Priority Groups are charged copayments for inpatient care, outpatient care, outpatient medication, and long-term care services. Only veterans in Priority Group 1 (those who have been rated 50% or more service-connected) and veterans who are deemed catastrophically disabled by a VA provider are never charged a copayment, even for treatment of a nonservice-connected condition. For veterans in other priority groups, VHA currently has four types of nonservice-connected copayments for which veterans may be charged: outpatient, inpatient, extended care services, and medication. Veterans in all priority groups are not charged copayments for a number of outpatient services, including the following: publicly announced VA health fairs; screenings and immunizations; smoking and weight loss counseling; telephone care; laboratory services; flat film radiology; and electrocardiograms.

For primary care outpatient visits, there is a $15 copayment charge and for specialty care outpatient visits, a $50 copayment. Veterans do not receive more than one outpatient copayment charge per day. That is, if the veteran has a primary care visit and a specialty care visit on the same day, the veteran pays only for the specialty care visit. For veterans required to pay an inpatient copayment charge, rates vary based upon whether the veteran is enrolled in Priority Group 7 or not. Veterans enrolled in Priority Group 8 and certain other veterans are responsible for the VA's full inpatient copayment, and veterans enrolled in Priority Group 7 and certain other veterans are responsible for paying 20% of the VA's inpatient copayment. Veterans in Priority Groups 1 through 5 do not have to pay inpatient or outpatient copayments. Veterans in Priority Group 6 may be exempt due to special eligibility for treatment of certain conditions. For veterans required to pay long-term care copayments, these charges are based on three levels of nonservice-connected care, including inpatient, non-institutional, and adult day health care. Actual copayments vary depending on the veteran's financial situation. For medication copayments, veterans are not billed if they have a service-connected disability rated 50% or greater, if they are former prisoners of war, or if their medications are related to certain eligibility exceptions. Veterans enrolled in Priority Groups 2 through 6 have a $960 calendar-year cap on the amount that they can be charged for these copayments. Veterans who are unable to pay VA's copayment charges may submit requests for assistance, including waivers, hardships, compromises, and repayment plans.[40]

Table 2. VA Reimbursement for Emergency Care

Service-Connected	Nonservice-Connected
The VA is required to pay or reimburse veterans for medical expenses incurred in non-VA facilities when all three of the following conditions apply:[a] (1) Delay would have been hazardous to the life or health of the veteran. (2) VA or other federal facilities were not feasibly available (or treatment had been refused). (3) The care was provided for: • a service-connected disability, • a nonservice-connected disability aggravating a service-connected disability, or • any disability of a veteran whose service-connected disability is total and permanent in nature.	The VA is required to pay or reimburse veterans for medical expenses incurred in non-VA facilities when all four of the following conditions apply: (1) Delay would have been hazardous to the life or health of the veteran. (2) VA or other federal facilities were not feasibly available. (3) The veteran has either: • no health coverage (e.g., private health insurance or Medicare) or • coverage that would only partially pay for the emergency treatment.[b] (4) In cases where the care was provided for a condition caused by an accident or work-related injury, all claims against a third party for payment have been exhausted without success.

Source: CRS Summary of 38 U.S.C. § 1728 and 38 U.S.C. § 1725.

a. Prior to the enactment of the Veterans' Mental Health and Other Care Improvements Act of 2008 (P.L. 110-387), the VA was not required to reimburse the non-VA facility for the cost of care after the point of stabilization. P.L. 110-387 mandated that the VA reimburse or pay for the reasonable value of treatment for any veteran who meets above eligibility criteria and defined "emergency treatment" as continuing until the veteran can be transferred safely to a VA or other federal facility, and the VA or other federal facility agrees to accept such a transfer.

b. Prior to the passage of the Veterans' Emergency Care Fairness Act (P.L. 111-137), a veteran who was enrolled in the VA's health care system was reimbursed for emergency treatment received at a non-VA hospital. However, the statute only permitted such VA reimbursement if the veteran had no other outside health insurance, no matter how limited that other coverage was. P.L. 111-137 would require the VA to pay for emergency treatment for a nonservice-connected condition if a third party is not responsible for paying for the full cost of care. The law also set two limitations on reimbursement as follows: (1) the VA is the secondary payer where a third-party insurer covers a part of the veteran's medical liability (e.g., his or her automobile insurance coverage, private health insurance, or Medicare Part A and Medicare Part B); and (2) the VA is only responsible for the difference between the amount paid by the third-party insurer and the VA allowable amount. Veterans would continue to be responsible for co-payments owed to the third-party insurer; if the veteran were responsible for copayments under a private health insurance or Medicare plan, then the veteran would still be liable to pay this (copayment rates and or coinsurance rates are set by the individual insurance policy or Medicare and not the VA). P.L. 111-137 clarifies that veterans are not liable for any remaining balance due to the provider after the third-party insurer and the VA have made their payments.

The VHA bills private health insurers for medical care, supplies, and prescriptions provided to veterans for their nonservice-connected conditions. While the VA cannot bill Medicare, it can bill Medicare supplemental health insurance carriers for covered services.[41] Veterans are not responsible for paying any remaining balance of the VA's insurance claim that is not paid or covered by their health insurance carrier. Any payment received by the VA is used to offset ''dollar for dollar'' a veteran's VA copayment responsibility.[42]

Table 3. Copayments for Health Care Services (CY2012)

	Inpatient care	**Outpatient care**	**Outpatient medication**	**Long-term care services**
	($10/day + $ $1,156 for first 90 days and $578 after 90 days; based on 365-day period)	**($15 Primary Care; $50 Specialty Care; $0 for x-rays, lab, immunizations, etc.)**	**($8 per 30-day supply; calendar year cap: $960 for Priority Groups 2-6; $9 for 30-day supply for Priority Groups 7 and 8)[a]**	**(Institutional nursing home care units, respite care, geriatric evaluation: $0-97 per day. Non-institutional respite care, geriatric evaluation, adult day healthcare: $15 per day; domiciliary care: $5 per day)**
Priority Group 1	NO	NO	NO	NO
Priority Group 2[b]	NO	NO	YES	NO
Priority Group 3[b]	NO	NO	YES	NO
Priority Group 4	NO	NO	NO	NO
Priority Group 5[c]	NO	NO	YES	YES
Priority Group 6[d]	NO	NO	NO	NO
Priority Group 7[e]	YES	YES	YES	YES
Priority Group 8[f]	YES	YES	YES	YES

Source: Table prepared by the Congressional Research Service based on information from the Department of Veterans Affairs.

Notes: "NO" means the veteran is *not* responsible for paying copayments. "YES" means the veteran *may be* liable for partial or full copayments.

a. For the period from July 1, 2010, through until December 31, 2012, the copayment amount for veterans in Priority Groups 2 through 6 is $8. There is an annual cap of $960 per calendar year. When veterans reach the annual cap, they continue to receive medications without making a co-payment. For veterans in Priority Groups 7 and 8 the copayment amount from July 1, 2010, through until December 31, 2012, is $9. There is no annual cap for these priority groups.

b. No medication copayments if medication is for a service-connected disability. Former POWs are exempt from all medication copayments.

c. No medication or long-term care copayments if veteran is in receipt of VA pension or has an income below applicable pension threshold.

d. Priority Group 6 are veterans claiming exposure to Agent Orange; veterans claiming exposure to environmental contaminants; veterans exposed to ionizing radiation; combat veterans within five years of discharge from the military; veterans who participated in Project 112/SHAD; veterans claiming military sexual trauma; and veterans with head and neck cancer who received nasopharyngeal radium treatment while in the military are subject to copayments when their treatment or medication is not related to their exposure or experience. The initial registry examination and follow-up visits to receive results of the examination are not billed to the health insurance carrier and are not subject to copayments. However, care provided that is not related to exposure, if it is nonservice-connected, will be billed to the insurance carrier and copayments can apply.

e. Priority Group 7a and 7c veterans have incomes above the VA Means Test threshold but below the Geographic Means Test threshold and are responsible for 20% of the inpatient copayment and 20% of the inpatient per diem copayment. The Geographic Means Test copayment reduction does not apply to outpatient and medication copayments, and veterans will be assessed the full applicable copayment charges.

f. Priority Group 8a and 8c veterans have incomes above the VA Means Test threshold and above the Geographic Means Test threshold. Veterans enrolled in these priority groups are responsible for the full inpatient copayment and the inpatient per diem copayment for care of their nonservice-connected conditions. Veterans in these priority groups are also responsible for outpatient and medication copayments for care of their nonservice-connected conditions.

Can the VA Bill Private Health Insurance?

The VA has the authority to bill most health care insurers for nonservice-connected care provided to veterans enrolled in the VA health care system.

The Consolidated Omnibus Budget Reconciliation Act of 1985 (P.L. 99-272), enacted into law in 1986, gave the VHA the authority to bill some veterans and most health care insurers for nonservice-connected care provided to veterans enrolled in the VA health care system to help defray the cost of delivering medical services to veterans.[43] This law also established means testing for veterans seeking care for nonservice-connected conditions.

Congress authorized the VHA to collect reasonable charges for medical care or services (including the provision of prescription drugs) from a third party to the extent that the veteran or the provider of the care or services would be eligible to receive payment from the third party for (1) a nonservice-connected disability for which the veteran is entitled to care (or the payment of expenses of care) under a health plan contract;[44] (2) a nonservice-connected disability incurred as a result of the veteran's employment and covered under a worker's compensation law or plan that provides reimbursement or indemnification for such care and services;[45] or (3) a nonservice-connected disability incurred as a result of a motor vehicle accident in a state that requires automobile accident reparations (no fault) insurance.[46] Similarly, the VHA can receive payments from Medicare supplemental coverage plans for nonservice-connected conditions for which the veterans receives care at VHA facilities.

Veterans are not responsible for paying any remaining balance of the VA's insurance claim not paid or covered by their health insurance. Any payment received by the VA is used to offset "dollar for dollar" a veteran's VA copayment responsibility.[47]

Can the VA Bill Medicare?

The VA is statutorily prohibited from billing Medicare[48] *in most situations.*

In general, Medicare is prohibited from reimbursing for any services provided by a federal health care provider unless

- the provider is determined by the Secretary of Health and Human Services (HHS) to be providing services to the public as a community institution or agency;
- the provider is providing services through facilities operated by the Indian Health Service (IHS);[49] or
- the services were provided in an emergency (in a hospital setting).

Medicare is also prohibited from making payments to any federal health care provider who is obligated by law or contract to render services at public expense.[50] Therefore, the VHA is statutorily prohibited from receiving Medicare payments for services provided to Medicare-covered veterans.[51] Although the legislative history does not indicate congressional intent for this decision, "a safe assumption to be drawn from the exclusion of Medicare [from paying for health care services provided through other federal entities] is that Congress wanted to avoid the unnecessary transfer of federal funds from Medicare to the VA when the money is all coming out of the same coffer."[52]

It should be noted that there is a narrow exception to this statutory prohibition of Medicare reimbursing the VHA. Under current law the VHA can be reimbursed by Medicare (notwithstanding any condition, limitation, or other provision in title XVIII of the Social Security Act) when the VA provides services to Medicare-covered individuals who are not eligible for care under Chapter 17 of Title 38 United States Code (U.S.C.)[53] and who are afforded VA care or services under a "sharing" agreement.[54]

APPENDIX. VA PRIORITY GROUPS AND THEIR ELIGIBILITY CRITERIA

The VA classifies veterans into eight enrollment Priority Groups based on an array of factors including (but not limited to) service-connected disabilities or exposures,[55] prisoner of war (POW) status, receipt of a Purple Heart or Medal of Honor, and income. The criteria for each Priority Group are summarized in **Table A-1**.

The eight Priority Groups fall into two broad categories. The first group is composed of veterans with service-connected disabilities or with incomes below an established means test. These veterans are regarded by the VA as "high priority" veterans, and they are enrolled in Priority Groups 1-6. Veterans enrolled in Priority Groups 1-6 include the following:

- veterans in need of care for a service-connected disability;
- veterans who have a compensable service-connected condition;
- veterans whose discharge or release from active military, naval, or air service was for a compensable disability that was incurred or aggravated in the line of duty;
- veterans who are former prisoners of war (POWs);
- veterans awarded the Purple Heart;
- veterans who have been determined by the VA to be catastrophically disabled;
- veterans of World War I;
- veterans who were exposed to hazardous agents (such as Agent Orange in Vietnam) while on active duty; and

- veterans who have an annual income and net worth below a VA-established means test threshold.

Table A-1. VA Priority Groups and Their Eligibility Criteria

Priority Group 1
Veterans with service-connected disabilities rated 50% or more disabling
Veterans determined by VA to be unemployable due to service-connected conditions
Priority Group 2
Veterans with service-connected disabilities rated 30% or 40% disabling
Priority Group 3
Veterans who are former POWs[a]
Veterans awarded the Purple Heart[b]
Veterans in receipt of the Medal of Honor[c]
Veterans whose discharge was for a disability that was incurred or aggravated in the line of duty
Veterans with service-connected disabilities rated 10% or 20% disabling
Veterans awarded special eligibility classification under Title 38, U.S.C., Section 1151, "benefits for individuals disabled by treatment or vocational rehabilitation"
Priority Group 4
Veterans who are receiving aid and attendance or housebound benefits
Veterans who have been determined by VA to be catastrophically disabled
Priority Group 5
Nonservice-connected veterans and noncompensable service-connected veterans rated 0% disabled whose annual income and net worth are below the established VA means test thresholds
Veterans receiving VA pension benefits
Veterans eligible for Medicaid benefits
Priority Group 6
Compensable 0% service-connected veterans
Mexican Border War veterans
Veterans solely seeking care for disorders associated with
• exposure to herbicides while serving in Vietnam; or
• ionizing radiation during atmospheric testing or during the occupation of Hiroshima and Nagasaki; or
• for disorders associated with service in the Gulf War; or
• for any illness associated with service in combat in a war after the Gulf War or during a period of hostility after November 11, 1998 as follows:

Table A-1. (Continued)

Priority Group 6
• Veterans discharged from active duty on or after January 28, 2003, who were enrolled as of January 28, 2008, and veterans who apply for enrollment after January 28, 2008, for five years post discharge
• Veterans discharged from active duty before January 28, 2003, who apply for enrollment after January 28, 2008, until January 27, 2011
Priority Group 7
Veterans who agree to pay specified copayments with income and/or net worth above the VA means test threshold and income below the VA national geographic income thresholds
Priority Group 8
Veterans who agree to pay specified copayments with income and/or net worth above the VA means test threshold and the VA national geographic threshold
Subpriority a: Noncompensable 0% service-connected and enrolled as of January 16, 2003, and who have remained enrolled since that date and/or placed in this subpriority due to changed eligibility status
Subpriority b: Noncompensable 0% service-connected and enrolled on or after June 15, 2009, whose income exceeds the current VA means test threshold or VA national geographic income thresholds by 10% or less
Subpriority c: Nonservice-connected veterans enrolled as of January 16, 2003, and who have remained enrolled since that date and/or placed in this subpriority due to changed eligibility status
Subpriority d: Nonservice-connected veterans enrolled on or after June 15, 2009, whose income exceeds the current VA means test threshold or VA national geographic income thresholds by 10% or less
Subpriority e: Noncompensable 0% service-connected veterans not meeting the above criteria
Subpriority g: Nonservice-connected veterans not meeting the above criteria

Source: Department of Veterans Affairs.

Notes: Service-connected disability means with respect to disability, that such disability was incurred or aggravated in the line of duty in the active military, naval or air service.

a. Veterans who are former prisoners of war (POWs) are in Priority Group 3. This began with the enactment of the Former Prisoner of War Benefits Act of 1981(P.L. 97-37) on August 14, 1981.

b. Veterans in receipt of a Purple Heart are in Priority Group 3. This began with the enactment of the Veterans Millennium Health Care and Benefits Act (P.L. 106-117) on November 30, 1999.

c. Veterans in receipt of the Medal of Honor are in Priority Group 3. This began with the enactment of the Caregiver and Veterans Omnibus Health Services Act of 2010 (P.L. 111-163) on May 5, 2010.

The VA looks at applicants' income and net worth to determine their specific priority category and whether they have to pay copayments for nonservice-connected care. In addition, veterans are asked to provide the VA with information on any health insurance coverage they have, including coverage through employment or through a spouse. The VA may bill these payers for treatment of conditions that are not a result of injuries or illnesses incurred or aggravated during military service.

The second group of veterans is composed of those who do not fall into one of the first six priority groups—primarily veterans with nonservice-connected medical conditions and with incomes and net worth above the VA-established means test threshold. These veterans are enrolled in Priority Groups 7 or 8.[56] **Table A-2** provides information on income thresholds for VA health care benefits.

Table A-2. National Income Thresholds for CY2012

Veterans with—	Free VA prescriptions and travel benefits for veterans with incomes of—	Free VA Heath Care for veterans with incomes of—
No dependents	$12,256 or less	$30,460 or less
1 dependent	$16,051 or less	$36,554 or less
2 dependents	$18,144 or less	$38,647 or less
3 dependents	$20,237 or less	$40,740 or less
4 dependents	$22,330 or less	$42,883 or less
For each additional dependent, add:	$2,093	$2,093

Source: Department of Veterans Affairs.

Notes: For geographic variations, see http://www.va.gov/healtheligibility/Library/AnnualThresholds.asp.

End Notes

[1] Department of Veterans Affairs, *FY2013 Budget Submission, Medical Programs and Information Technology Programs*, Volume 2 of 4, February 2012, p. 1A-3.

[2] U.S. Department of Veterans Affairs, *FY 2011 Performance and Accountability Report*, Washington, DC, November 15, 2011, p. I-31. Established on January 3, 1946, as the Department of Medicine and Surgery by P.L. 79-293, succeeded in 1989 by the Veterans Health Services and Research Administration, and renamed the Veterans Health Administration in 1991.

[3] Adam Oliver, "The Veterans Health Administration: An American Success Story?" *The Milbank Quarterly*, vol. 85, no. 1 (March 2007), pp. 5-35.

[4] For a detailed discussion of "promised benefits," see CRS Report 98-1006, *Military Health Care: The Issue of "Promised" Benefits*, by David F. Burrelli.

[5] Barbara Sydell, "Restructuring the VA Health Care System: Safety Net, Training and Other Considerations," National Health Policy Forum, Issue Brief no. 716, March 1998.

[6] U.S. Congress, House Committee on Veterans Affairs, *Veterans' Health Care Eligibility Reform Act of 1996*, report to accompany H.R. 3118, 104th Cong. 2nd sess., H.Rept. 104-690, p. 2.

[7] A service-connected disability is a disability that was incurred or aggravated in the line of duty in the U.S. Armed Forces (38 U.S.C. §101 (16)). The VA determines whether veterans have service-connected disabilities, and for those with such disabilities, assigns ratings from 0% to 100% based on the severity of the disability. Percentages are assigned in increments of 10% (38 C.F.R. §§4.1-4.31).

[8] H.Rept. 104-690, p. 5.

[9] Ibid., p. 6.

[10] Ibid., p. 5.

[11] A service-connected disability is a disability that was incurred or aggravated in the line of duty in the U.S. Armed Forces (38 U.S.C. §101 (16)). The VA determines whether veterans have service-connected disabilities, and for those with such disabilities, assigns ratings from 0% to 100% based on the severity of the disability. Percentages are assigned in increments of 10% (38 C.F.R. §§4.1-4.31).

[12] Veterans meeting certain income criteria may be eligible to enroll in the VA without a service-connected condition.

[13] Generally, persons enlisting in one of the Armed Forces after September 7, 1980, and officers commissioned after October 16, 1981, must have completed two years of active duty or the full period of their initial service obligation to be eligible for VA health care benefits. Servicemembers discharged at any time because of service-connected disabilities are not held to this requirement.

[14] A veteran with an "other than honorable" discharge or "bad conduct" discharge may still retain eligibility for VA health care benefits for disabilities incurred or aggravated during service in the military. For more information on the nature of discharge requirements, see CRS Report R42324, "*Who is a Veteran?"—Basic Eligibility for Veterans' Benefits*, by Christine Scott.

[15] For those servicemembers who are called to duty multiple times, this will be the most recent discharge date. Generally, returning combat veterans are assigned to Priority Group 6, unless eligible for a higher Priority Group, and are not charged copays for medication and/or treatment of conditions that are potentially related to their combat service. At the end of the five-year period, veterans enrolled in Priority Group 6 may be re-enrolled in Priority Group 7 or 8, depending on their service-connected disability status and income level, and may be required to make copayments for nonservice-connected conditions. The above criteria apply to National Guard and Reserve personnel who were called to active duty by federal executive order and served in a theater of combat operations after November 11, 1998.

[16] A service-connected disability is a disability that was incurred or aggravated in the line of duty in the U.S. Armed Forces (38 U.S.C. §101 (16)). The VA determines whether veterans have service-connected disabilities, and for those with such disabilities, assigns ratings from 0% to 100% based on the severity of the disability. Percentages are assigned in increments of 10% (38 C.F.R. §§4.1-4.31).

[17] A service-connected disability is a disability that was incurred or aggravated in the line of duty in the U.S. Armed Forces (38 U.S.C. §101 (16)). The VA determines whether veterans have service-connected disabilities, and for those with such disabilities, assigns ratings from 0%

to 100% based on the severity of the disability. Percentages are assigned in increments of 10% (38 C.F.R. §§4.1-4.31).

[18] 38.U.S.C. §101(24); 38 C.F.R. §3.6(c).

[19] VA Form 10-10EZ is available at https://www.1010ez.med.va.gov/sec/vha/1010ez/. Veterans do not need to apply for enrollment in the VA's health care system if they fall into one of the following categories: veterans with a service-connected disability rated at 50% or more (percentages of disability are based upon the severity of the disability, and those with a rating of 50% or more are placed in Priority Group 1); veterans for whom less than one year has passed since the veteran was discharged from military service for a disability that the military determined was incurred or aggravated in the line of duty, but the VA has not yet rated; or the veteran is seeking care from the VA only for a service-connected disability (even if the rating is only 10%).

[20] H.Rept. 104-690, p. 4.

[21] For example, veterans who may have been exposed to Agent Orange during the Vietnam War or veterans who may have diseases potentially related to service in the Gulf War may be eligible to receive care.

[22] 38 C.F.R. §17.36 (d)(3)(iv) (2009).

[23] For more information on the VA family caregiver program, see http://www.caregiver.va.gov/support_benefits.asp.

[24] Hearing aids and eyeglasses are part of the standard medical package for veterans meeting either of the following criteria: (1) any veteran with a service-connected condition rated 50% or more on one or more disabilities or based on Individual Unemployability or (2) veterans needing care for a service-connected condition.

[25] A detailed listing of the VHA's standard medical benefits package is available at 38 C.F.R. §17.38.

[26] 38 C.F.R. §17.38.

[27] 38 C.F.R. §17.38; and Department of Veterans Affairs, Veterans Health Administration, *Health Care Services for Women Veterans*, VHA Handbook 1330.01, May 21, 2010.

[28] Department of Veterans Affairs, "VA Dental Insurance Program," 77 *Federal Register* 12517, March 1, 2012.

[29] 38 C.F.R. §17.149, and Department of Veterans Affairs, *Prescribing Hearing Aids and Eyeglasses*, VHA Directive2008-070, October 28, 2008.

[30] Activities of Daily Living (ADLs) generally refer to activities such as bathing, getting in and out of a bed or chair, eating, dressing, walking across the room, and using the toilet.

[31] This section is based on Carol J. Sheets and Heather Mahoney-Gleason, "Caregiver Support in the Veterans Health Administration: Caring For Those Who Care," *GENERATIONS – Journal of the American Society on Aging*, vol. 34, no. 2 (Summer 2010), pp. 92-98.; U.S. Department of Veterans Affairs, Office of Care Coordination, Supporting Veterans' Caregivers: A Frequently Asked Questions Guide, November 29, 2006, pp. 15-18.; and U.S. Congress, House Committee on Veterans' Affairs, Subcommittee on Health, *Legislative Hearing on H.R. 1293, H.R. 1197, H.R. 1302, H.R. 1335, H.R. 1546, H.R. 2734, H.R. 2738, H.R. 2770, H.R. 2898 and Draft Discussion Legislation*, 111th Cong., 1st sess., June 18, 2009 (Washington: GPO, 2009), pp. 57-58.

[32] Activities of Daily Living (ADLs) generally refer to activities such as bathing, getting in and out of a bed or chair, eating, dressing, walking across the room, and using the toilet. Instrumental Activities of Daily Living (IADLs) may include activities such as shopping for groceries, light housework, preparing hot meals, using the telephone, taking medications, and managing money.

[33] The CRC program is authorized under 38 U.S.C. §1730.

[34] 38 U.S.C. §§1703,1725, and 1728.

[35] Department of Veterans Affairs, Veterans Health Administration, *Audit of Non-VA Inpatient Fee Care Program*, Report No: 09-03408-227, Washington, DC, August 18, 2010, p. 1.

[36] Under current law, "emergency treatment" is defined as medical services furnished, in the judgment of the VA Secretary (1) when VA or other federal facilities are not feasibly available and an attempt to use them beforehand would not be reasonable; (2) when such services are rendered in a medical emergency of such nature that a prudent layperson reasonably expects that delay in seeking immediate medical attention would be hazardous to life or health; and (3) until such time as the veteran can be transferred safely to a VA facility (38 U.S.C. §1725(f)(1)).

[37] 38 U.S.C. §1728.

[38] 38 U.S.C. §1725.

[39] The VA classifies veterans into eight enrollment Priority Groups based on an array of factors including (but not limited to) service-connected disabilities or exposures, prisoner of war (POW) status, receipt of a Purple Heart or Medal of Honor, and income. The criteria for each Priority Group are summarized in the **Appendix**.

[40] U.S. Congress, House Committee on Veterans' Affairs, Subcommittee on Health, *Identifying the Causes of Inappropriate Billing Practices by the U.S. Department of Veterans Affairs*, 111th Cong., 1st sess., October 15, 2009(Washington: GPO, 2010), p. 43.

[41] 38 U.S.C. §1729.

[42] U.S. Congress, House Committee on Veterans' Affairs, Subcommittee on Health, *Identifying the Causes of Inappropriate Billing Practices by the U.S. Department of Veterans Affairs*, 111th Cong., 1st sess., October 15, 2009(Washington: GPO, 2010), p. 43.

[43] Veterans' Health-Care and Compensation Rate Amendments of 1985 (P.L. 99-272).

[44] 38 U.S.C. §1729(a)(2)(D), and 38 C.F.R. §17.101(a)(1)(i).

[45] 38 U.S.C. §1729(a)(2)(A), and 38 C.F.R. §17.101(a)(1)(ii).

[46] 38 U.S.C. §1729(a)(2)(B), and 38 C.F.R. §17.101(a)(1)(III).

[47] U.S. Congress, House Committee on Veterans' Affairs, Subcommittee on Health, *Identifying the Causes of Inappropriate Billing Practices by the U.S. Department of Veterans Affairs*, 111th Cong., 1st sess., October 15, 2009 (Washington: GPO, 2010), p. 43.

[48] "Medicare is a federal insurance program that pays for covered health care services of qualified beneficiaries." CRS Report R40425, *Medicare Primer*, coordinated by Patricia A. Davis.

[49] In 1976, Congress authorized Medicare and Medicaid payments for services delivered in Indian health facilities(whether operated by the IHS or Tribes) through amendments to the Social Security Act made in the Indian HealthCare Improvement Act of 1976 (P.L. 94-437) (IHCIA). This was permanently authorized by the Patient Protection and Affordable Care Act (PPACA; P.L. 111-148). According to the *Centers for Medicare and Medicaid Services American Indian and Alaska Native Strategic Plan 2010–2015*: "this entitlement funding was expected to provide critical resources to improve the quality of health care for American Indians and Alaska Natives and to reduce the health status disparities. There is a provision in the IHCIA that Medicaid and Medicare revenues shall not offset congressional appropriations for the IHS, so that the total amount of funding for Indian health care would increase and not merely be shifted from one funding stream to another"(available at http://www.cmsttag.org/docs/CMS%20Strategic%20Plan%20-%20June%2010,%202009%20FINAL.pdf).

[50] 42 U.S.C. §§1395f(c), 1395n(d), 1395f(a).

[51] 42 U.S.C §1395f(c), and 38 U.S.C. §1729(i)(1)(B)(i).

[52] United States v. Blue Cross & Blue Shield of Maryland, Inc., 989 F.2d 718, 727 n. 5 (4th Cir.).

[53] Chapter 17 of Title 38 U.S.C. details the eligibility criteria as well as programs relating to the provision of medical care, and nursing home care, among other things, for veterans and their eligible dependents.

[54] 38 U.S.C. §8153(d). A sharing agreement is a written contract that allows VHA to buy, sell, or exchange health care resources and services with non-VA facilities. VHA could enter into noncompetitive sharing agreements with affiliated institutions (such as affiliated medical schools) and other entities associated with these affiliated institutions (such as university hospitals).

[55] For example, veterans who may have been exposed to Agent Orange during the Vietnam War or veterans who may have diseases potentially related to service in the Gulf War may be eligible to receive care.

[56] The VA considers a veteran's previous year's total household income (both earned and unearned income, as well as his/her spouse's and dependent children's income). Earned income is usually wages received from working. Unearned income includes interest earned, dividends received, money from retirement funds, Social Security payments, annuities, and earnings from other assets. The number of persons in the veterans' family will be factored into the calculation to determine the applicable income threshold. 38 C.F.R. §17.36(b)(7) (2009).

In: Veteran's Health Care
Editor: Claude Da Costa
ISBN: 978-1-62417-371-4

Chapter 2

"WHO IS A VETERAN?" — BASIC ELIGIBILITY FOR VETERANS' BENEFITS*

Christine Scott

SUMMARY

A broad range of benefits are offered to veterans of the U.S. Armed Forces and to certain members of their families by the U.S. Department of Veterans Affairs (VA). Among these benefits are various types of financial assistance, including monthly cash payments to disabled veterans, health care, education, and housing benefits. Basic criteria must be met to be eligible to receive any of the benefits administered by the VA.

For a former service member to receive certain VA benefits, the person must have active U.S. military service for a minimum period of time and meet nature of discharge requirements. Some members of the National Guard and reserve components have difficulty meeting the active duty and length of service requirements. However, a member of the National Guard or reserve components who is activated for federal military service and serves the full period of activation is considered a veteran for purposes of VA benefits.

* This is an edited, reformatted and augmented version of the Congressional Research Service Publication, CRS Report for Congress R42324, dated January 23, 2012.

The GI Bill Improvement Act of 1977 (P.L. 95-202) recognized the service of one group of civilians, the Women's Air Forces Service Pilots, as active service for benefits administered by the VA, and it also established that the Secretary of Defense could determine that service for the Armed Forces by a group of civilians, or contractors, be considered active service for benefits administered by the VA.

This report examines the basic eligibility criteria for VA administered veterans' benefits, including the issue of eligibility of members of the National Guard and reserve components.

INTRODUCTION

A broad range of benefits are offered to veterans of the U.S. Armed Forces and to certain members of their families by the U.S. Department of Veterans Affairs (VA). Among these benefits are various types of financial assistance, including monthly cash payments to disabled veterans, health care, education, and housing benefits. Basic criteria must be met to be eligible to receive any of the benefits administered by the VA.

This report focuses upon the basic eligibility/entitlement requirements for former servicemembers for veterans' benefits administered by the VA. Certain VA benefits are available to current servicemembers, and the eligibility requirements for those benefits are not a component of this report.

The VA uses a two-step process to evaluate claims for benefits. First, the claimant must demonstrate that he or she is *eligible*. That is, the claimant must prove that he or she is a bona fide veteran and verify certain related matters. In this sense, the eligibility relates to the veteran's general qualification(s) for the benefit(s). Second, the veteran must prove *entitlement* to the particular benefit being sought.[1]

WHO IS A VETERAN?

To be eligible for most VA benefits, the claimant must be a veteran or, in some circumstances, the survivor or the dependent of a veteran. By statute, a "veteran" is defined as a "person who served in the active military, naval, or air service, and who was discharged or released therefrom under conditions other than dishonorable."[2]

In evaluating the evidence to determine whether the applicant is a "veteran" for the purposes of VA benefits, the VA relies upon military department service records. The VA is bound by information that the service documents contain.[3] Generally speaking, the VA findings will be in accord with the information contained in the applicant's military service records.[4]

Such records may include an original military service record; a copy issued by the military service with the certification that it is a true document; or a copy submitted by an accredited agent, attorney, or service representative with special training, who certifies that it is a copy of an original military service document or a copy of a copy of such a document.[5] In addition to meeting these criteria, the document must contain data regarding the length, time, and character of the service, and the VA must believe that the document is genuine and accurate.[6] If the claimant does not provide the requisite documentation or other evidence, or the submitted documentation does not meet the requirements, the VA must seek to verify the applicant's military service directly from the appropriate military service.[7]

Active Service

An applicant must have "active military, naval, or air service" to be considered a veteran for most VA benefits.[8] However, not all types of service are considered active military service for this purpose.[9]

In general, active service means full-time service, other than active duty for training, as a member of the Army, Navy, Air Force, Marine Corps, Coast Guard, or as a commissioned officer of the Public Health Service, the Environmental Science Services Administration or the National Oceanic and Atmospheric Administration, or its predecessor, the Coast and Geodectic Survey.

Active service also includes a period of active duty for training during which the person was disabled or died from an injury or disease incurred or aggravated in the line of duty[10] and any period of inactive duty for training during which the person was disabled or died from an injury incurred or aggravated in the line of duty or from certain health conditions incurred during the training.[11]

Additional circumstances of service, and whether they are deemed to be active military service, are set out in law.[12] For example, if on authorized travel to and from the performance of active duty training or inactive duty for training, a person is disabled or dies while proceeding directly to or returning from such duty, the duty will be considered to be active duty for training or inactive duty for training.[13]

The determination of whether a claimant has met the "active service" requirement may not be a simple process. It is possible that the claimant and the VA may have to scrutinize the claimant's service record(s) to determine whether the claimant's service fits into one of the many categories of active service, or whether an exception has been made for his or her service, so that it is considered to be active service for the purposes of veterans' benefits. In addition, a claimant may have more than one period of service, which may further complicate the determination.

Length of Service

Prior to September 8, 1980, there was no minimum length of service necessary to be considered a veteran for most VA benefits. However, for an individual who enlisted after September 8, 1980, there are now certain minimum length of service requirements. The general requirement is either 24 months of continuous active duty or the "full period" for which the servicemember was called or ordered to active duty.[14]

Several exceptions exist to this general rule. For example, service-connected disability compensation benefits are exempt from the minimum active duty requirements. Thus, a veteran with a disease or injury incurred during active service should almost always be able to receive service-connected compensation for his or her condition or disability.[15] Other exceptions to the minimum service requirements include claims for VA life insurance benefits,[16] hardship discharges,[17] and persons retired or separated from service because of a service-related disability.[18]

If the former servicemember does not fall within the 24 months of active duty or the "full period" of active duty, or within one of the statutory exceptions, then the veteran has not completed a minimum period of active duty and is "not eligible for any benefit under Title 38, United States Code or under any law administered by the Department of Veterans Affairs based on that period of active service."[19]

Discharge Criteria

The statutory definition of "veteran" requires that the individual be discharged or released from military service "under conditions other than dishonorable."[20] There are currently five types of discharges issued by the military services: (1) honorable discharge (HD), (2) discharge under honorable conditions (UHC) or general discharge (GD), (3) discharge under other than honorable conditions (UOTHC) or undesirable discharge (UD), (4) bad conduct discharge (BCD), and (5) dishonorable discharge (DD).[21]

The language of the statute does not precisely match the current categories of the discharges, and the VA often determines on a case-by-case basis whether the claimant's discharge satisfies any of the criteria and which category of discharge applies. In most cases, the VA considers honorable discharges and discharges under honorable conditions to fall within the "conditions other than dishonorable" category, and will usually qualify the claimant as a veteran under the first step of the eligibility test.[22] Usually, honorable and general discharges qualify a veteran for most benefits.[23]

A bad conduct discharge from a special court-martial and other discharges made under other than honorable conditions may or may not disqualify the claimant from being considered a veteran for purposes of benefits eligibility.[24] In the case of such a discharge, the VA will make a special "character of service determination," based on the particular facts in the claimant's case. On this basis, the VA will determine whether the veteran was separated from service under "dishonorable conditions" or under "other than dishonorable conditions." The VA will review the entire period of the claimant's enlistment(s) to assess the quality of the service and to determine whether it is sufficient to deserve the award of veterans' benefits.[25] If a claimant has served more than one period of enlistment, he or she may have two or more different discharge categories.

Dishonorable and bad conduct discharges issued by general courts-martial may bar VA benefits. Veterans in prison and parolees may be eligible for certain VA benefits and must contact the VA to determine eligibility. VA benefits will not be provided to any veteran or dependent wanted for an outstanding felony warrant.

Certain exceptions permit the award of VA benefits, even if the character of the discharge would ordinarily bar VA benefits. For example, if it is determined that the claimant was insane at the time of the offense leading up to the discharge, the claimant may be granted VA benefits. There does not need to be a direct connection between the insanity and the misconduct.[26]

Whether the Military Service Was during a Time of War[27]

All military service is classified as either wartime or peacetime service. Whether a veteran has served during a time of war may impact his or her potential VA benefits. For example, the Improved Pension benefit for low-income veterans who are either elderly or non-service-connected disabled veterans, is only for veterans with wartime service.[28]

Congress has set out the periods of "wartime" for the purposes of veterans' benefits.[29] To be considered to have "served during wartime" by the VA, a veteran does not have to have served in an actual combat zone, but during the specified periods of war set out below. Those time periods not designated by Congress as "wartime" are considered to be "peacetime." If a veteran served his or her duty partly during wartime and partly during peacetime, the veteran would meet the "wartime" criteria if he or she served 90 consecutive days, at least one day of which occurred during a period designated as wartime.

Following is a list of those periods of "wartime" designated by Congress:

- *Indian Wars*—January 1, 1817, through December 31, 1898[30]
- *Spanish-American War*—April 21, 1898, through July 4, 1902[31]
- *Mexican Border Period*—May 19, 1916, though April 5, 1917[32]
- *World War I*—April 6, 1917, through November 11, 1918; extended to April 1, 1920; by regulation extended to July 1, 1921, under certain specific conditions[33]
- *World War II*—December 7, 1941, through December 31, 1946; extended to July 25, 1947[34]
- *Korean Conflict*—June 27, 1950, through January 31, 1955[35]
- *Vietnam Era*—August 5, 1964, through May 7, 1975[36]
- *Persian Gulf War*—August 2, 1990, through a date to be prescribed by Presidential proclamation or law[37]

NATIONAL GUARD AND RESERVE

Two particular elements of the criteria to be a veteran—"active duty" and "length of service"— are often difficult for members of the National Guard and the reserve components to meet. As a result, these servicemembers, having not met the statutory threshold criteria for "veteran," are often not eligible for VA benefits.

In many cases, members of the Guard and the reserves may not have fulfilled the "active duty" requirement. Members of the Guard and reserves who have never been activated for federal active duty military service, and consequently have not served on regular federal active duty, do not meet the active duty requirement for the definition of a veteran for VA benefits.

For other National Guard and reserve members, the two requirements may be met at the same time. An example of this situation would be a Guard or reserve member who was activated for federal military service and served in the Persian Gulf for 12 months. At the end of the activation period, the servicemember would be considered to have served on active duty for that period of time. Serving for the full period of activation also meets the minimum length of service requirement to be a veteran. Otherwise, Guard and reserve duty may not be considered "active duty" for benefits unless the servicemember performing this duty was disabled or died from a disease or injury incurred or aggravated in the line of duty.[38]

Although many National Guard and reserve members may not appear to be eligible "veterans" for the purposes of VA benefits, certain exceptions and special circumstances may exist, which add to the complexity of the eligibility determination. For example, under certain conditions Guard and reserve members may be eligible for education benefits (through the Reserve Educational Program or the Post-9/11 GI Bill) and home loans from the VA (with six years of service in the Selected Reserves or National Guard). As each servicemember's military service may be different, and therefore may fit within certain case categories or exceptions, eligibility is usually determined by the VA on a case-by-case basis after reviewing the individual servicemember's military service records.

CIVILIAN GROUPS

The GI Bill Improvement Act of 1977 (P.L. 95-202) recognized the service of one group of civilians, the Women's Air Forces Service Pilots, as active service for benefits administered by the U.S. Department of Veterans Affairs. In addition, P.L. 95-202 provided that the Secretary of Defense could determine that service for the Armed Forces by a group of civilians, or contractors, be considered active service for benefits administered by the VA.

Based on the provisions of P.L. 95-202,[39] the Secretary of Defense established that the Secretary of the Air Force would develop and maintain the process to determine if the wartime employment of certain groups of individuals is considered "active duty" military service for the purpose of receiving certain veterans benefits. If these groups of individuals are considered to be "active duty" by the Secretary, they are eligible to receive certain benefits, including health care.[40]

Regulations implementing P.L. 95-202 specify which groups the Secretary has determined were employed in "active duty" service.[41] The regulations also established the Department of Defense Civilian/Military Service Review Board and Advisory Panel to review each application for "active duty" status.[42] Following its review, the board issues a written recommendation to the Secretary as to whether the applicant group should be considered "active duty" for the purposes of the act. The Secretary makes the final decision, based upon the recommendation of the board. Pursuant to this procedure, various groups of persons have been accorded "active duty" status. Among the successful applicants were Women's Air Forces Service Pilots (WASPs), Signal Corps Female Telephone Operators Unit (World War I), Engineer Field Clerks (World War I), Male Civilian Ferry Pilots (World War II), and other groups of employees with war-related occupations.[43] At this time, all of the successful applicants have been civilian groups associated with World War I and World War II.

The regulations concerning the designation of "active duty" status have undergone revision over the years. Changes and clarification to the regulations implemented in 1989 "stem from a Federal Court determination [*Schumacher v. Aldridge*][44] that the Department of Defense had failed to clarify factors and criteria in their implementing directive concerning P.L. 95-202."[45] The 1989 regulations remain in effect.

End Notes

[1] For example, to be entitled to receive disability compensation, a veteran must provide sufficient evidence of certain elements (e.g., current diagnosis, medical evidence of an in-service occurrence, and link between the in-service occurrence and the current disability).

[2] 38 U.S.C. § 101(2); 38 C.F.R. § 3.1(d).

[3] Venturella v. Gober, 10 Vet. App. 340, 341-342 (1977); Duro v. Derwinski, 2 Vet. App. 530, 532 (1992).

[4] 38 C.F.R. § 3.203.

[5] 38 C.F.R. § 3.203(a)(1). See CRS Report RS21282, *Military Service Records and Unit Histories: A Guide to Locating Sources*, by Julissa Gomez-Granger and Anne Leland.

[6] 38 C.F.R. § 3.203(a)(2), (3).
[7] Duro, 2 Vet. App. at 532.
[8] 38 U.S.C. § 101(2); 38 C.F.R. § 3.12(a).
[9] For example, National Guard and Reserve duty may not be considered active service unless an individual performing this duty was disabled or died from a disease or injury incurred or aggravated in the line of duty. (38 U.S.C. § 101(24); 38 C.F.R. § 3.6(a)).
[10] Active duty for training is a tour of active duty that is used for training members of reserve and other components to fill the Armed Forces during time of war or national emergency. Active duty for training has been determined to mean (1) full-time duty for training performed by Reservists (38 U.S.C. § 101(22)(A); 38 C.F.R. § 3.6(c)(1)); (2) full-time duty for training purposes as a commissioned officer in the Reserved Corps of the Public Health Service (38 U.S.C. § 101(22)(B); 38 C.F.R. § 3.6(c)(2)); (3) full-time training duty by members of the Air or Army National Guard of any state (38 U.S.C. § 101(22)(C); 38 C.F.R. § 3.6(c)(3)); (4) duty by members of the Senior ROTC program on field training or a practice cruise (38 U.S.C. § 101 (22)(D); 38 C.F.R. § 3.6(c)(4)); and (5) authorized travel to and from duty for training (38 U.S.C. § 101(22)(E); 38 C.F.R. § 3.6(c)(6)).
[11] 38 U.S.C. § 101(24). Inactive duty for training has been defined to mean (1) duty, other than full-time duty, for Reservists (38 U.S.C. § 101(23)(A); 38 C.F.R. § 3.6(d)(1)); (2) other duties authorized for Reservists performed on a voluntary basis (38 U.S.C. § 101(23)(B); 38 C.F.R. § 3.6(d)(2)); (3) training (other than active duty for training) by a member of, or applicant for membership in, Senior ROTC (38 U.S.C. § 101(23)(C); 38 C.F.R. § 3.6(d)(3)); and (4) for the members of the Air or Army National Guard of any state, such training means duty other than full-time duty (38 U.S.C. § 101(23); 38 C.F.R. § 3.6(d)(4)).
[12] 38 U.S.C. §§ 101, 106.
[13] 38 U.S.C. § 106(d); 38 C.F.R. § 3.6(e).
[14] 38 U.S.C. § 5303A(b); 38 C.F.R. § 3.12a(a)(1).
[15] 38 U.S.C. § 5303A(b)(3)(C); 38 C.F.R. § 3.12a(d)(4).
[16] 38 U.S.C. § 5303A(b)(3)(E); 38 C.F.R. § 3.12a(d)(5).
[17] 38 U.S.C. § 5303A(b)(3)(A); 38 C.F.R. § 3.12a(d)(1).
[18] 38 U.S.C. § 5303A(b)(3)(B); 38 C.F.R. § 3.12a(d)(2).
[19] 38 U.S.C. § 5303A(b)(1); 38 C.F.R. § 3.12a(b).
[20] 38 U.S.C. § 101(2); 38 C.F.R. § 3.12(a).
[21] Barton F. Stichman et al., *Veterans Benefits Manual*, at § 2.2.1 (Cited to afterward as "Veterans Benefits Manual").
[22] Ibid.
[23] Ibid.
[24] Ibid.
[25] Ibid.
[26] 38 U.S.C. § 5303(b).
[27] See CRS Report RS21405, *U.S. Periods of War and Dates of Current Conflicts*, by Barbara Salazar Torreon.
[28] 38 U.S.C. § 1521(j).
[29] 38 U.S.C. § 101 (6)-(11); 38 C.F.R. § 3.2.
[30] See 38 C.F.R. § 3.2(a).
[31] 38 U.S.C. § 101(6); 38 C.F.R. § 3.2(b).
[32] 38 U.S.C. § 101(30); 38 C.F.R. § 3.2(h).
[33] 38 U.S.C. § 101(7); 38 C.F.R. § 3.2(c).
[34] 38 U.S.C. § 101(8); 38 C.F.R. § 3.2(d).
[35] 38 U.S.C. § 101(9); 38 C.F.R. § 3.2(e).
[36] 38 U.S.C. § 101(29); 38 C.F.R. § 3.2(f). Military personnel who served in the Republic of Vietnam between February 28, 1961, and May 7, 1975, are also considered to have served during the Vietnam Era.

[37] 38 U.S.C. §§ 101(33), 1501(4); 38 C.F.R. §§ 3.2(I), 3.3(a)(3), 3.17, 3.54(a)(3)(viii). At the present time, no termination date has been established.

[38] 38 U.S.C. § 101(21)(A); 38 C.F.R. § 3.6(a). Inactive duty would include duty other than full-time duty, such as weekend assignments or part-time details.

[39] 38 U.S.C. § 106 note.

[40] See 38 C.F.R. § 3.7.

[41] 32 C.F.R. § 47. See 38 C.F.R. § 3.7 for those groups that have been so designated.

[42] The applications are usually submitted by representatives of the employment group.

[43] 38 C.F.R. § 3.7.

[44] 665 F.Supp. 41 (D.D.C. 1987).

[45] 54 *Fed.* Reg. 39,991 (September 29, 1989).

In: Veteran's Health Care
Editor: Claude Da Costa

ISBN: 978-1-62417-371-4

Chapter 3

HEALTH CARE FOR DEPENDENTS AND SURVIVORS OF VETERANS*

Sidath Viranga Panangala

SUMMARY

The Civilian Health and Medical Program of the Department of Veterans Affairs (CHAMPVA) is primarily a fee-for-service program that provides reimbursement for most medical care for certain eligible dependents and survivors of veterans rated permanently and totally disabled from a service-connected condition. This report provides an overview of CHAMPVA and includes a series of questions and answers about the program.

OVERVIEW

The Veterans Health Administration (VHA) of the Department of Veterans Affairs (VA) provides health care services to veterans who meet certain eligibility requirements. The VHA is primarily a direct service provider of primary care, specialized care, and related medical and social support services to veterans though an integrated health care system. In 1973,

* This is an edited, reformatted and augmented version of a Congressional Research Service publication, CRS Report for Congress RS22483, from www.crs.gov, prepared for Members and Committees of Congress, dated February 18, 2010.

Congress established the Civilian Health and Medical Program of the Department of Veterans Affairs (CHAMPVA) as a means of providing health care services to dependents and survivors of certain veterans.[1] As stated in the House report accompanying P.L. 93-82:

> The nation has long recognized that the widow and children of a veteran who dies ofserviceconnected disease or injury or of a veteran who has a service-connected total disability are in a special category and deserving of substantial compensation and assistance in return for the sacrifice the family has made. This recognition has been shown in title 38 programs which provide for death compensation benefits, home loans, and educational assistance benefits for wives, widows, and war orphans. Failure to provide for the medical care of such individuals is an oversight which should be corrected.[2]

CHAMPVA primarily is a fee-for-service program that provides reimbursement for most medical care for certain eligible dependents and survivors of veterans rated permanently and totally disabled from a service-connected condition.[3] CHAMPVA is a cost-sharing program that reimburses providers and facilities a determined allowable amount, minus patient co-pay and deductible. CHAMPVA was designed to provide medical care in a manner similar to the care provided to certain eligible beneficiaries under the Department of Defense (DOD) TRICARE program (see the description below). The number of beneficiaries enrolled in CHAMPVA has grown over the years. From FY2001 through FY2009, enrollment grew by 248%—from 96,500 to 336,300 beneficiaries (see *Figure 1*). The 2001 expansion of CHAMPVA eligibility to certain individuals aged 65 years and older has contributed to the increase in enrollment. Moreover, there has been an increase in enrollment of dependents and spouses of certain Vietnam-era veterans with service-connected disabilities. This increase in Vietnam-era CHAMPVA sponsorship has occurred as aging Vietnam-era veterans with service-connected disabilities experience a worsening of symptoms and a change in disability status. Once a veteran becomes VA-rated permanently and totally disabled for a service-connected disability, the veteran's spouse and dependents are then eligible to enroll in CHAMPVA.

Funding for CHAMPVA is provided through the VHA's Medical Services account.[4] As shown in *Table 1,* spending for CHAMPVA grew steadily in the past eight years. Between FY2002 and FY2009, CHAMPVA expenditures increased by 336%, while the number of unique users increased by only 187% during the same period. These data imply an increased average cost per patient from approximately $2,495 per patient in FY2002 to $3,791 per patient in FY2009.

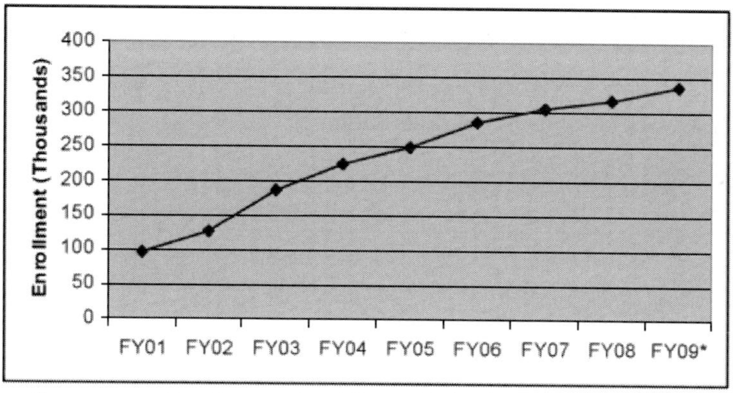

Source: Chart prepared by Congressional Research Service (CRS), based on data from the Department of Veterans Affairs.

* These are the estimated enrolled beneficiaries for FY2009.

Figure 1. CHAMPVA-Enrolled Beneficiaries, FY2001-FY2009.

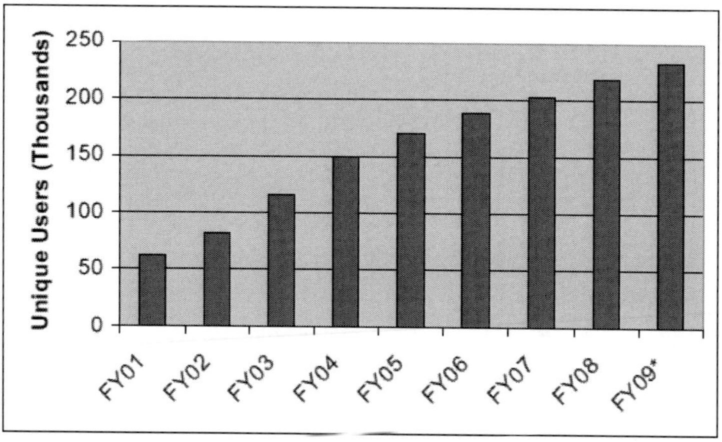

Source. Chart prepared by Congressional Research Service (CRS), based on data from the Department of Veterans Affairs.

* These are the estimated enrolled beneficiaries for FY2009.

Figure 2. CHAMPVA Unique Users, FY2002-FY2009.

A demographic shift in CHAMPVA enrollees from less expensive younger beneficiaries to more expensive aging beneficiaries, in addition to the general inflation of medical costs, has contributed to the increase in CHAMPVA expenditures.

Table 1. CHAMPVA Expenditures, FY2002-FY2009 ($ in millions)

	FY2002 Actual	FY2003 Actual	FY2004 Actual	FY2005 Actual	FY2006 Actual	FY2007 Actual	FY2008 Actual	FY2009 Actual
Expenditures	$203.1	$318.2	$454.5	$565.5	$656.9	$712.2	$794.0	$885.2

Source: Table prepared by Congressional Research Service (CRS), based on data from the U.S. Department of Veterans Affairs, Congressional Budget Submissions (FY2004-11), Medical Programs.

The next section provides answers to frequently asked questions about the program.

QUESTIONS AND ANSWERS[5]

Who Is Eligible to Receive CHAMPVA Benefits?

Eligibility for CHAMPVA requires inclusion in one of the following categories:[6]

- the individual is the spouse or child of a veteran who has been rated permanently and totally disabled for a service-connected disability;
- the individual is the surviving spouse or child of a veteran who died from a VA-rated service-connected disability;
- the individual is the surviving spouse or child of a veteran who was at the time of death rated permanently and totally disabled from a service-connected disability; or
- the individual is the surviving spouse or child of a military member who died on active duty, not due to misconduct (in most cases, these family members are eligible under TRICARE, not CHAMPVA).

What Happens if a CHAMPVA-Eligible Spouse Divorces or Remarries?

CHAMPVA eligibility is terminated by divorce or annulment of marriage to the qualifying veteran. CHAMPVA has specific eligibility rules for widows. When a CHAMPVA-eligible widow remarries, eligibility is terminated if the marriage occurs before the age of 55. As of February 4, 2003, a CHAMPVA-eligible widow who remarries at age 55 or older remains eligible for CHAMPVA. If a CHAMPVA-eligible widow under the age of 55 remarries, and the remarriage is later terminated, the widow is again eligible for CHAMPVA.

When Does a Child Lose Eligibility?

In general, eligibility for CHAMPVA is lost when either a child (other than a helpless child)[7] turns 18, unless enrolled in an accredited school as a full-time student; a child, who has been a full-time student, turns 23 or loses full-time student status; a child marries; or a stepchild no longer lives in the household of the sponsor.

What Is the Difference Between CHAMPVA and TRICARE?

Before distinguishing between the two programs, it is important to make the distinction between a veteran and a military retiree. Title 38 of the United States Code defines a "veteran" as a person who has been discharged under conditions other than dishonorable from active military, naval, or air service.[8] All military retirees, by definition, are veterans. However, to be considered a "military retiree," an individual generally must have spent at least 20 years on active duty in the armed services. CHAMPVA is a comprehensive program run by the VA for eligible family members of veterans rated permanently and totally disabled for a service-connected disability or the family members of veterans who died from a VA-rated service-connected disability. The sponsoring veteran does not receive services through CHAMPVA, as he or she is eligible to receive services through the VA. Dependents of military retirees are not eligible for CHAMPVA, and must apply for benefits through TRICARE. TRICARE is a health care program run by the DOD for families of active duty military service members, families of service members who died while on active duty, and retired military service men, women, and their families, regardless of their disability status. TRICARE has no disability criteria required for eligibility.[9]

What Is the Relationship of CHAMPVA and Medicare?

Under section three of the Veterans' Survivors Benefits Improvement Act of 2001, referred to as CHAMPVA for Life (P.L. 107-14), CHAMPVA benefits were expanded to those over the age of 65 in the following circumstances. CHAMPVA is the secondary payer for beneficiaries with Medicare coverage.

- If a beneficiary turns 65 before June 5, 2001, and only receives Medicare Part A, the beneficiary is eligible for CHAMPVA without having to purchase Medicare Part B coverage.
- If a beneficiary turns 65 before June 5, 2001, and receives both Medicare Part A and Part B, the beneficiary must retain both parts to be eligible for continued CHAMPVA as secondary coverage.
- If a beneficiary turns 65 on or after June 5, 2001, the beneficiary must be enrolled in Medicare Parts A and B to be eligible for CHAMPVA.
- Enrollment in Medicare Part D is not required to become or remain eligible for CHAMPVA.
- Individuals aged 65 or older not entitled to Medicare Part A retain CHAMPVA eligibility.

What Happens if the Beneficiary Has Other Health Insurance?

By law, CHAMPVA is generally the secondary payer for beneficiaries having any other form of health insurance. The primary health insurance company is billed first, and then beneficiaries submit an explanation of benefits (EOB) for additional reimbursement by CHAMPVA. The exception is for beneficiaries with Medicaid, beneficiaries receiving care under the State Victims of Crime Compensation Program, or beneficiaries with a CHAMPVA supplementary insurance policy. In those cases, CHAMPVA is the first payer.[10]

What Medical Benefits Are Available to Eligible Beneficiaries?

The CHAMPVA program covers most health care services and supplies that are determined to be medically necessary, including inpatient and outpatient care, prescription drugs, mental health services, and skilled nursing care. By law, CHAMPVA is required to provide health care benefits that are similar to the DOD's TRICARE program. Chiropractic services, routine eye examinations, hearing aids, and most dental benefits are excluded from both the federal CHAMPVA and TRICARE programs.[11] In late 2008, benefits were expanded to include any non-dental prostheses and removed the exclusion from coverage of enuretic (bed-wetting) devices.[12]

Certain types of care require advance approval, commonly know as preauthorization. Generally, a CHAMPVA beneficiary should ask a provider if the provider will accept a CHAMPVA beneficiary. This is known as "accepting assignment." What that means is the provider will bill the VA directly for covered services, items and supplies. They will be paid the "allowable charge." Doctors or providers who agree to accept assignment cannot try to collect more than the CHAMPVA deductible and cost share amounts from the beneficiary. If provider does not accept assignment, the CHAMPVA beneficiary is responsible for paying the annual deductible, the cost share amount (copay), and any provider-billed amount that exceeds our total allowable amount.

For care that is not covered by CHAMPVA, the beneficiary has to pay the full bill.[13] For example, with very few exceptions, dental care is not a covered benefit. Currently, preauthorization is required for

- durable medical equipment,
- hospice services,
- mental health/substance abuse services,
- organ and bone marrow transplants, and
- dental procedures that are directly related to covered medical conditions.

What Is the CHAMPVA Payment Structure?

CHAMPVA is a cost-sharing program that reimburses at rates comparable to the Medicare and TRICARE programs. CHAMPVA has an outpatient deductible of $50 per person and $100 per family per calendar year. After the deductible is reached, CHAMPVA pays 75% of the allowable amount, and the beneficiary pays 25% of the total amount.[14] The patient typically pays the cost share at the time the service is provided, unless the beneficiary has another health insurance plan. In cases where a beneficiary has another form of health insurance, CHAMPVA is the secondary payer (with the exception of the circumstances outlined in question five), and pays the lesser of either 75% of the allowable amount after the deductible or the rest of the billed charges. There is a $3,000 cap on cost sharing per CHAMPVA-eligible family. There is also an exception to the payment scheme outlined here for instances in which medical services are rendered through VA facilities participating in the CHAMPVA In-house Treatment Initiative (CITI).[15]

What Is the CHAMPVA In-House Treatment Initiative (CITI)?

The CITI is a voluntary program for CHAMPVA beneficiaries that provides medical care through local VA facilities on a space-available basis. Beneficiaries receiving care at the VA through the CITI program are not required to pay a deductible or participate in cost sharing. No extra enrollment is necessary to participate in the CITI program; the beneficiary simply has to determine if the local VA is a participating facility. The majority of VA facilities are CITI participants. It is important to emphasize that care is delivered based on the availability of space. Beneficiaries on Medicare or who have an HMO plan as their primary insurance are not eligible for the CITI program.

How Are CHAMPVA Claims Processed?

All CHAMPVA claims are processed through the VA Health Administration Center (HAC) in Denver, Colorado. Claims can be submitted by either the provider or the beneficiary, with each case requiring a different set of forms. All claims must be filed within one year after the date of service. For inpatient care, the claim must be filed within one year of the discharge date, and all payments will be made to the hospital regardless of which party submits the billing. Claims submitted after the one-year deadline will be denied. As of 2009, the ceiling on durable medical equipment (DME) was raised to $2,000 to facilitate the administrative claims process and to accurately reflect the current costs of medical equipment.[16]

End Notes

[1] Veterans Health Care Expansion Act of 1973 (P.L. 93-82).

[2] U.S. Congress, Committee on Veterans' Affairs, Veterans Health Care Expansion Act of 1973, report to accompany H.R. 9048, 93rd Congress, first session, H.Rept. 93-368 (Washington: GPO, 1973).

[3] The term "service-connected" means, with respect to disability, that such disability was incurred or aggravated in the line of duty in the active military, naval, or air service. VA determines whether veterans have service-connected disabilities, and for those with such disabilities, assigns ratings from 0 to 100% based on the severity of the disability. Percentages are assigned in increments of 10%.

[4] For detailed information on VHA appropriations, see CRS Report R40737, Veterans Medical Care: FY2010 Appropriations, by Sidath Viranga Panangala.

[5] This part was drawn from: Department of Veterans Affairs Health Administration Center, CHAMPVA Handbook, at http://www.va.gov/hac/forbeneficiaries/champva/handbook/chandbook.pdf and http://www4.va.gov/hac/ forbeneficiaries/champva/champva.asp

[6] 38 U.S.C. § 1781; 38 C.F.R. § 17.270-17.278.

[7] A helpless child is established after a fact-based analysis completed by a VA Regional Office determines the child to be permanently incapable of self-support by the age of 18. See 38 C.F.R. § 3.356 and http://www.va.gov/hac/ forbeneficiaries/champva/handbook/chandbook.pdf.

[8] 38 U.S.C. § 101.

[9] For further information on TRICARE, see CRS Report RL33537, Military Medical Care: Questions and Answers, by Don J. Jansen. For specific provisions, see http://www.TRICARE.osd.mil; relevant regulations are at 32 C.F.R. § 199.

[10] 38 C.F.R. § 17.275.

[11] 38 C.F.R. § 17.272.

[12] Department of Veterans Affairs, "Civilian Health and Medical Program of the Department of Veterans Affairs (CHAMPVA): Expansion of Benefit Coverage for Prostheses and Enuretic Devices; Miscellaneous Provisions," 73 Federal Register 65552, November 4, 2008.

[13] Department of Veterans Affairs Health Administration Center. Fact Sheet 01-16 for Outpatient Providers and Office Managers. p. 1.

[14] An allowable amount is the maximum payment that is authorized by the VA for a covered medial service or supply.

[15] 38 C.F.R. § 17.274.

[16] Department of Veterans Affairs, "(CHAMPVA): Preauthorization of Durable Medical Equipment," 74 Federal Register 31373, July 1, 2009.

In: Veteran's Health Care
Editor: Claude Da Costa
ISBN: 978-1-62417-371-4

Chapter 4

VETERANS HEALTH CARE: VETERANS HEALTH ADMINISTRATION PROCESSES FOR RESPONDING TO REPORTED ADVERSE EVENTS*

United States Government Accountability Office

The Honorable Patty Murray
Chairman
Committee on Veterans' Affairs United States Senate

The Honorable Bob Filner
Ranking Member
Committee on Veterans' Affairs House of Representatives

The Department of Veterans Affairs' (VA) Veterans Health Administration (VHA) operates one of the largest health care delivery systems in the United States, providing care to more than 6 million veterans annually. Organized into 21 Veterans Integrated Service Networks, VHA's health care system includes 152 Veterans Affairs medical centers (VAMC) nationwide that offer a variety of outpatient, residential, and inpatient services.[1] These

* This is an edited, reformatted and augmented version of The United States Government Accountability Office publication, GAO-12-827R, dated August 24, 2012.

health care services are delivered by physicians, dentists, and other providers and range from routine examinations to complex surgical procedures.

During the course of providing health care services, adverse events[2]—clinical incidents that may pose the risk of injury to a patient as the result of a medical intervention or lack of an appropriate intervention, such as a missed or delayed diagnosis, rather than that patient's underlying medical condition[3]—may occur, resulting in potential harm to veterans. They are required to be reported to appropriate VAMC staff through each facility's incident reporting system,[4] or through other channels, such as anonymous phone calls or e-mails to VAMC staff, such as the patient safety manager or risk manager, according to officials.[5] VHA policy requires that appropriate action be taken to evaluate reported adverse events.[6] Once an adverse event has been evaluated, the VAMC may take actions that include correcting system or process issues and taking actions against individual clinicians when warranted. Specifically, actions taken against individual clinicians following adverse events may include adverse actions—ranging from admonishments[7] to termination of employment; as well as actions taken to limit a clinician's clinical privileges, such as the reduction or revocation of privileges.[8] Staff remediation activities, such as refresher training and proctoring, can be employed when adverse actions or limiting a clinician's privileges are not deemed necessary.

Recent adverse events have raised questions about the quality of care provided to veterans by VAMCs, and whether lessons learned at one VAMC are being translated into systemwide improvements. In response, members of Congress have raised questions as to the processes VHA has in place to respond to adverse events at VAMCs and take appropriate action, when needed, to address problems found within the VHA health care system. You asked us to describe how VHA responds to reported adverse events within its health care system. In this report, we describe VHA's processes for responding to reported adverse events within its health care system. In future work, we will examine the implementation of these processes at VAMCs. To describe VHA's processes for responding to reported adverse events, we reviewed and analyzed documentation that contains policy and guidance for these processes,[9] including VA and VHA directives and handbooks. Specifically, we examined processes that enable VAMCs to determine the cause of an adverse event and assessed the characteristics of these processes. We also reviewed VHA's processes for taking action to help prevent an adverse event from recurring, such as correcting process or system deficiencies, using remediation approaches such as retraining and proctoring, and taking adverse actions against clinicians responsible for an adverse event. We also interviewed officials from VHA's Office of Quality, Safety, and Value, about issues related to quality, safety, and risk management and adverse actions.[10] Our review was limited to VHA physicians and dentists, hereafter referred to as clinicians, as they are the primary types of licensed clinicians[11] that practice independently at VAMCs. Furthermore, our review was limited to describing VHA's processes for responding to adverse events, rather than all quality-of-care issues, such as those that did not rise to the level of an adverse event.

We conducted this performance audit from April 2012 through August 2012 in accordance with generally accepted government auditing standards. Those standards require that we plan and perform the audit to obtain sufficient, appropriate evidence to provide a reasonable basis for our findings and conclusions based on our audit objectives. We believe that the evidence obtained provides a reasonable basis for our findings and conclusions based on our audit objectives.

VHA Generally Allows VAMCs Discretion in Responding to Reported Adverse Events

Through its policy and guidance, VHA has outlined processes that enable VAMCs to respond to reported adverse events that occur.[12] VHA generally grants individual VAMCs discretion on choosing which process to use. Specifically, VAMCs conduct an initial review to determine how best to respond to an adverse event. According to VHA officials, if the circumstances that led to an adverse event are clear, based on a VAMC's initial review, VAMCs can take immediate corrective action. If the circumstances that led to an adverse event need to be examined further, VAMCs are given discretion to use one or more of the following four processes: (1) root cause analysis, (2) peer review, (3) clinical care review, and (4) administrative investigation board.[13] Because VAMCs generally have discretion in which of these processes they use, different VAMCs that experience similar adverse events may not use the same processes to respond to them. Nonetheless, each process has certain purposes and limitations. For example, some of these processes may be used to examine a clinician's actions as they relate to an adverse event, while others may be used to examine whether a systems or process issue exists. Furthermore, information collected through two of these processes—clinical care reviews and administrative investigation boards—can be used to inform actions against clinicians; information collected using root cause analyses and peer reviews cannot be used to support such actions, because information collected under those processes is protected and confidential, under federal law.[14] Based on the nature of an adverse event and the information gleaned through a particular review process, a VAMC may decide to conduct multiple types of reviews, as appropriate.[15] Figure 1 shows VHA's four processes for responding to reported adverse events.

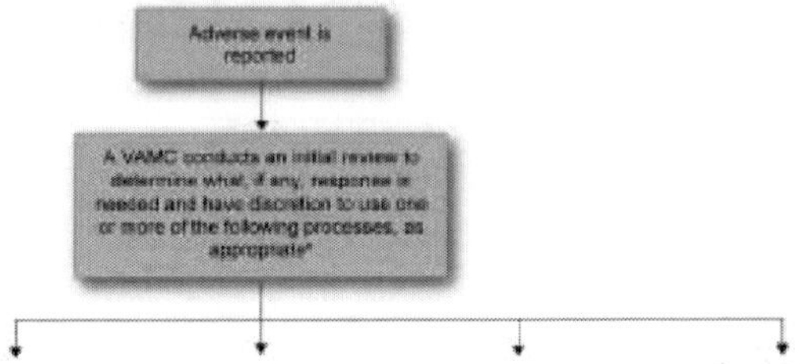

Purpose	Root cause analysis	Peer review	Clinical care review	Administrative investigation board
Examine a clinician's actions as they relate to an adverse event		•	•	•
Examine whether a systems or process issue exists	•			•
Use and Limitations				
Information is protected and confidential, and cannot be used to inform any adverse action against a clinician	•	•		
Information can be used to inform adverse action against a clinician			•	•
Information can be used to make systems or process changes	•			•

Source: GAO analysis of VHA information.

Figure 1. VHA's Processes for Responding to Reported Adverse Events at VAMCs.

Root Cause Analysis

If the VAMC's initial review of an adverse event finds that there is a risk to the safety of veterans, a root cause analysis may be required by VHA policy. To determine if a root cause analysis is required, the patient safety manager[16] evaluates the event using VHA's "safety assessment code matrix." This scoring tool measures safety risk based on the severity of an adverse event and its likelihood of occurrence on a scale of one (lowest risk) to three (highest risk). For example, an adverse event with a score of three is one that has the potential to result in death or permanent loss of function regardless of its likelihood of occurrence.[17] As directed by VHA policy, adverse events with a score of three always require a root cause analysis, either individual or aggregated.[18]

To conduct a root cause analysis, a VAMC director convenes a multidisciplinary team, which includes appropriate subject matter experts from the VAMC, such as clinicians and quality management staff. The team attempts to identify the systemic causes for an adverse event by determining what factors contributed to the event and why those factors occurred. Furthermore, the team identifies changes that could be made in systems and processes, such as through the development of new processes that would improve performance and reduce the risk of the adverse event recurring. For example, in a case that identified the root causes of a VAMC's failure to properly sterilize a piece of reusable medical equipment, a root cause analysis was used to examine whether instructions for cleaning the equipment were clear, whether sufficient training was provided to staff, and to develop steps to address these root causes.

Information gleaned through a root cause analysis may be used to make systems or process changes within a specific VAMC or VHA's health care system more broadly. The details of a root cause analysis are protected and confidential under federal law, meaning that they are protected from disclosure within and outside of VHA and cannot be used to take any adverse action or privileging action against clinicians.[19] According to officials, the lessons learned from the root cause analysis process may be used to provide lessons to the larger healthcare system.

Peer Review

If the VAMC's initial review or a root cause analysis finds there is a need to determine whether a clinician's actions associated with an adverse event were clinically appropriate—that is, whether another clinician with similar expertise would have taken similar action—a VAMC may initiate a peer review.[20]

During a peer review, the peer reviewer—a clinician or group of clinicians with similar expertise to the clinician involved in the incident being reviewed—evaluates the actions of the clinician under review to make an initial determination of whether the clinician should have taken different action when providing patient care. At the conclusion of this evaluation, the peer reviewer preliminarily rates the clinician's actions as one of the following:

- Level 1, at which the most experienced, competent clinician would have managed the case in a similar manner;
- Level 2, at which the most experienced, competent clinician might have managed the case differently; or
- Level 3, at which the most experienced, competent clinician would have managed the case differently.

If the peer reviewer initially rates the clinician's actions at Level 2 or 3, the clinician's case is referred to the VAMC's peer review committee—a multidisciplinary group of clinicians and/or other clinical staff members, such as nurses—which reviews the clinician's actions. Clinicians under review are given the opportunity to appear before the peer review committee or submit written comments to explain their actions. The peer review committee either validates the initial rating or assigns a higher or lower final rating of Level 1, 2, or 3.[21] The final rating is reported to the clinician's supervisor and, when appropriate, the VAMC director. The clinician's supervisor provides the clinician feedback based on the peer review committee's findings. According to officials, clinicians may be offered training to help them improve clinical proficiency, as determined to be appropriate by the supervisor. However, as is the case for root cause analyses, information obtained through peer reviews is protected and confidential and cannot be used to inform an adverse action or privileging action against a clinician.

Clinical Care Review

According to VHA officials, if the initial review finds there is a need to determine whether a clinician's actions associated with an adverse event were clinically appropriate, VAMCs have discretion to conduct a clinical care review. Through a clinical care review, a clinician's competency—his or her ability to provide an appropriate standard of care—is reviewed, to determine what type of action, if any, should be taken.[22] In addition, the peer review process can trigger a subsequent clinical care review. Each VAMC is required by VHA to establish its own criteria for review, such as triggers—that is, the number of Level 1, 2, and 3 peer reviews pertaining to an individual clinician over the course of a designated period of time that result in a clinical care review. For example, at one VAMC, three Level 3 peer reviews within a 6-month period would trigger a clinical care review.

According to VHA officials, to the extent that concerns about a clinician's competency are verified through a clinical care review, VAMCs may decide to initiate a focused professional practice evaluation or pursue privileging action[23] against the clinician. According to VHA officials, through a focused professional practice evaluation, a clinician is given an opportunity to improve his or her clinical competence over a period of time as determined by the VAMC director. At the discretion of the VAMC director, this evaluation can include progressive training or proctoring aimed at helping the clinician improve clinical competence.[24] Should concerns about clinical competence remain at the conclusion of a focused professional practice evaluation, a VAMC may then pursue privileging action against the clinician. VA policy affords clinicians due process prior to any privileging action. VAMCs are required to report physicians and dentists whose privileges are reduced, revoked, or surrendered while under investigation to the National Practitioner Data Bank,[25] which tracks information including privileging actions, as well as to report to appropriate state licensing boards, which may use this information to take action against the clinicians' medical licenses, including revoking, restricting, or suspending the license.[26]

Administrative Investigation Board

If the initial review finds that an investigation is warranted to determine whether an adverse event was the result of a clinician's professional misconduct or potential systemic deficiencies related to VHA policies or procedures, a VAMC director may convene an administrative investigation board.[27] A VAMC director also may choose to convene an administrative investigation board if a root cause analysis or peer review indicates an adverse event may have been the result of a clinician's professional misconduct. If this occurs, any ongoing root cause analysis or peer review is terminated or suspended until the administrative investigation board is concluded. Furthermore, the same individuals involved in conducting a root cause analysis or peer review may not be members of administrative investigation boards examining the same issues. Because any information collected through a root cause analysis or peer review is protected and confidential under federal law and cannot be used to take adverse action, information must be recollected when convening an administrative investigation board—that is, the board cannot use information collected and reviewed during the root cause analysis or peer review in its investigation.

Once an administrative investigation board is convened, it collects and analyzes evidence, such as sworn witness testimony and documentation, related to the allegation under investigation. Additionally, the board may obtain all available documents, records, and other information that are material to the scope of the investigation, including VHA policies, employee personnel records, and e-mail correspondence.[28] The board analyzes the collected evidence and develops the findings and conclusions of the investigation, including whether any allegations investigated were substantiated.

The board documents results—evidence, findings, conclusions, and any recommendations—in an investigation report that is forwarded to the VAMC director, who reviews the report to verify that the board sufficiently investigated the matter.[29] The VAMC director may accept the report or may ask the board to further investigate the matter, clarify the information in the investigation report, or both. VA considers an investigation to be complete once the VAMC director certifies the investigation report.

VAMC directors may use administrative investigation boards' findings to inform their decisions of whether to take adverse action against a clinician and, if so, which type of action to pursue.[30] Although VA policy provides guidance on the type of adverse action that should be taken in the case of certain offenses, the VAMC director has discretion over what adverse action, if any, to pursue. If adverse action is taken against a clinician, a standardized process for taking such action must be followed, which is defined by VA policy and is dependent on the type of action being taken. In addition to, or instead of, taking adverse action against an individual clinician, action may be taken to address systemic deficiencies related to policy or procedure found to have contributed to adverse events identified through an administrative investigation board. Furthermore, a VAMC director may decide to take nonadverse action, such as counseling or training, to expand a clinician's knowledge about VHA policies and procedures or clinical standards.

Agency Comments

VA provided us with comments on a draft of this report. In its comments, VA expressed concerns about specific language in the draft report that the department believed was either incomplete or could mislead the reader, and provided technical comments to address its concerns. We maintain that the draft report accurately described VHA's processes for responding to reported adverse events as explicitly described in VA and VHA policies and communicated to us by VHA officials. We have incorporated VA's technical comments as appropriate. However, because these technical comments did not require material changes to the draft report, we did not reprint them.

Debra A. Draper
Director, Health Care

End Notes

[1] In addition, VHA provides outpatient care at more than 800 community-based outpatient clinics.

[2] For the purposes of this report, the term "adverse event" includes "close calls." A close call is an event that could have the potential to result in an adverse event, but did not due to chance or timely intervention. Close calls receive the same level of scrutiny as adverse events that result in actual patient injury. Adverse events may or may not be attributable to an error made by a clinician, such as falls unrelated to patient care.

[3] An example of an adverse event is the improper sterilization of medical equipment that was reported at a VAMC, which led to veterans potentially being exposed to infectious diseases. VHA also responds to incidents in addition to adverse events, such as incidences of reported thefts or conflicts between employees. Such incidences are not considered adverse events and are not the subject of this report.

[4] Each VAMC maintains its own incident reporting system, which is used by VAMC staff to report information on adverse events.

[5] When an adverse event results in serious injury or death, or is reasonably expected to result in serious injury, VAMCs are required to disclose the event to the affected veteran or their representative through a formal process known as institutional disclosure. Institutional disclosure is generally carried out by a member of the VAMC's leadership and involves providing the veteran or their representative with information on how to seek compensation. For adverse events that cause less significant harm, VAMCs are required to disclose the event to the affected veteran or his or her representative through an informal process known as clinical disclosure.

[6] In addition to identifying and reporting adverse events, VAMCs have a quality management program in place that allows them to identify and respond to other quality-of-care issues that may not rise to the level of an adverse event.

[7] An admonishment is a written statement of censure given to an employee for a minor act of misconduct, such as repeated tardiness.

[8] Clinical privileges refer to authority granted to a clinician by a VAMC to provide patient care in the facility. Such privileges are limited by the individual clinician's license, experience, and competence. Some clinicians are VA employees, who may be employed on a full-time or part-time basis under permanent or temporary appointments, and others are contractors. Actions taken against individual clinicians may vary based on the employment status of the clinician. For example, for possible incompetence or professional misconduct by a contractor, VA may terminate the contract, thereby automatically revoking the contractor's medical staff appointment and clinical privileges, rather than taking adverse action or privileging action as can be done in cases of potential misconduct for employees.

[9] Both VA and VHA handbooks and directives contain policies and guidance regarding the processes for addressing an adverse event.

[10] The Office of Quality, Safety, and Value is charged with enhancing the quality, safety, reliability, and value of clinical and business systems throughout VA by enabling enterprisewide approaches to compliance, risk awareness, and continuous improvement.

[11] VA requires its physicians and dentists to possess at least one full, active, current, and unrestricted license to practice medicine or dentistry with limited exceptions, such as a state license limited on the basis of not meeting state residence requirements or a state-granted institutional license permitting full, unrestricted clinical practice at a specific VA health care facility.

[12] We use the term "processes" to refer to all policies, procedures, and processes governing VHA's response to reported adverse events.

[13] Additionally, in certain cases, such as when a veteran files a complaint to VA's Office of Inspector General or VHA's Office of the Medical Inspector, either of these entities may decide to independently investigate the adverse event.

[14] Under federal law, records and documents created as part of VHA's medical quality assurance program are confidential and privileged and may only be disclosed under limited circumstances. See 38 U.S.C. § 5705; 38 C.F.R. §§ 17.500-17.511. VHA's medical quality assurance program consists of systematic healthcare reviews carried out by or for VHA for the purposes of improving the quality of medical care or improving the utilization of healthcare resources in VHA medical facilities. The root cause analysis and peer review processes are part of VHA's medical quality assurance program, and as such, documents generated through these processes are confidential and privileged. 38 U.S.C. § 5705 was enacted out of concern that, unless clinicians could be assured that their remarks and assessments about possible problems with the healthcare services they deliver or one of their peers delivers to patients would be kept confidential, the necessary level of candor would be lost. Additionally, if the negative results from quality assurance activities were publicly available, the clinicians under review may be guarded or uncooperative during the review process. See 126 Cong. Rec. S10918 (Aug. 6, 1980) (excerpting S. Rep. No. 96-876).

[15] For example, a VAMC may decide to conduct an administrative investigation board and a root cause analysis in response to an adverse event to examine both a clinician's actions and to examine whether a systems or process issue exists.

[16] Each VAMC has a patient safety manager whose responsibilities include facilitating the root cause analysis process.

[17] An example of an adverse event with a score of two is one that has the potential to result in the permanent impairment of a bodily function which may occur occasionally—that is, several times over a 1- to 2-year period. An example of an adverse event with a score of one is one that has the potential to result in an increased length of stay for a veteran, which may occur occasionally.

[18] An aggregated root cause analysis collects information from multiple similar adverse events to conduct a single root cause analysis. An aggregated root cause analysis is required with several types of incidents: patient falls, adverse drug events, and missing patients. When not required, VAMCs have discretion to conduct aggregated root cause analyses for adverse events that receive a score of one or two.

[19] 38 U.S.C. § 5705; 38 C.F.R. §§ 17.500-17.511.

[20] While VHA policy requires that peer reviews be considered under certain circumstances, such as when a VAMC becomes aware of a veteran's death, each VAMC maintains a facility-

specific peer review policy that describes the specific circumstances under which a peer review is to be considered or required.

[21] VHA policy also requires the peer review committee to provide a secondary review of a representative sample of Level 1 peer reviews as a way to evaluate the peer review process in general.

[22] Each VAMC determines under which circumstances a clinical care review is appropriate and how it is to be conducted. For example, during a clinical care review, a clinician's supervisor may select a number of cases to review to help determine whether the clinician provided an appropriate standard of care.

[23] The VAMC director is the final authority for all privileging decisions. This decision must be based on the recommendations of the appropriate service chief(s), chief of staff, and/or the Executive Committee of the Medical Staff. Clinicians are given the right to reply to a proposed privileging action prior to a final action. Once the VAMC director makes a final determination on a privileging action, the clinician is entitled to a fair hearing by a panel of peers. If a privileging action is sustained following a fair hearing, clinicians have the right to appeal the decision to the network director, who may ultimately sustain or reverse the privileging action. In addition, adverse action, such as termination of employment, may be taken in conjunction with, or instead of privileging action, depending on the nature of the adverse event.

[24] Proctoring refers to an objective evaluation of a clinician's clinical competence by a peer.

[25] The National Practitioner Data Bank is an information clearinghouse that collects and releases all licensure actions or other negative actions taken against clinicians, including malpractice payments.

[26] If a clinician resigns or retires prior to privileging action being taken, VHA policy requires that he or she be reported to the National Practitioner Data Bank and appropriate state licensing boards.

[27] Administrative investigation boards also may be convened by authorities senior to a VAMC director within the network or VHA. Administrative investigation boards also are used to investigate matters besides adverse events, such as allegations of wrongdoing that involve nonclinical matters or matters involving potential systems deficiencies related to a VHA policy or procedure. See GAO, VA Administrative Investigations: Improvements Needed in Collecting and Sharing Information, GAO-12-483 (Washington, D.C.: Apr. 30, 2012).

[28] Some information relevant to an investigation, such as patient medical records, may not be available to the board, or may be subject to specific restrictions on disclosure or use.

[29] Upon convening an administrative investigation board, the VAMC director may authorize the board to provide recommendations for corrective actions. However, the board is prohibited from recommending a specific level or type of adverse action, such as termination or suspension. Although an administrative investigation board may provide recommendations for corrective actions, the VAMC director is not required to implement them.

[30] Although an administrative investigation board's findings may be used by a VAMC director to inform adverse actions, the board is not involved in determining such actions.

In: Veteran's Health Care
Editor: Claude Da Costa

ISBN: 978-1-62417-371-4

Chapter 5

VA HEALTH CARE: WEAKNESSES IN POLICIES AND OVERSIGHT GOVERNING MEDICAL SUPPLIES AND EQUIPMENT POSE RISKS TO VETERANS' SAFETY*

United States Government Accountability Office

ABBREVIATIONS

AEMS/MERS	Automated Engineering Management System/ Medical Equipment Reporting System
GIP	Generic Inventory Package
HIV	Human Immunodeficiency Virus
MQAS	Management Quality Assurance Service
OIG	Office of Inspector General
RME	reusable medical equipment
SOP	standard operating procedure
SPD	Supply, Processing, and Distribution
VA	Department of Veterans Affairs
VAMC	Veterans Affairs medical center
VHA	Veterans Health Administration

---

* This is an edited, reformatted and augmented version of The United States Government Accountability Office publication, Report to Congressional Requesters, GAO-11-391, dated May 2011.

VISN	Veterans Integrated Service Network

WHY GAO DID THIS STUDY

Department of Veterans Affairs (VA) clinicians use expendable medical supplies—disposable items that are generally used one time—and reusable medical equipment (RME), which is designed to be reused for multiple patients. VA has policies that VA medical centers (VAMC) must follow when purchasing such supplies and equipment, tracking these items at VAMCs, and reprocessing—that is, cleaning, disinfecting, and sterilizing—RME. GAO was asked to evaluate purchasing, tracking, and reprocessing requirements in VA policies and (2) VA's oversight of VAMCs' compliance with these requirements. GAO reviewed VA policies and selected two purchasing requirements, two tracking requirements, and two reprocessing requirements. At the six VAMCs GAO visited, GAO interviewed officials and reviewed documents to examine the adequacy of the selected requirements to help ensure veterans' safety. GAO also interviewed officials from VA headquarters and from six Veterans Integrated Service Networks (VISN), which oversee VAMCs, and obtained and reviewed documents regarding VA's oversight.

WHAT GAO RECOMMENDS

GAO is making several recommendations for VA to address the inadequacies identified in selected tracking and reprocessing requirements and the weaknesses in its oversight over selected purchasing and reprocessing requirements. VA concurred with these recommendations.

WHAT GAO FOUND

GAO found that the VA tracking and reprocessing requirements selected for review are inadequate to help ensure the safety of veterans who receive care at VAMCs. GAO did not identify inadequacies in selected VA purchasing requirements that may create potential risks to veterans' safety. GAO found the following:

- Tracking requirements. Because VA does not require VAMCs to enter information about certain expendable medical supplies and RME in their facilities into VA's inventory management systems, VAMCs may have incomplete inventories of these items. This, in turn, creates potential risks to veterans' safety. For example, in the event of a manufacturer recall involving these items, VAMCs may be unable to readily determine whether the items are in their facilities and should be removed and not used when providing care to veterans.
- Reprocessing requirements. Although VA requires VAMCs to develop device-specific training for staff on how to correctly reprocess RME, VA has not specified the types of RME for which this training is required. VA has also provided conflicting guidance to VAMCs on how to develop this training. This lack of clarity may have contributed to delays in developing the required training. Without appropriate training on reprocessing, VAMC staff may not be reprocessing RME correctly, which poses potential risks to the safety of veterans. VA headquarters officials told GAO that VA has plans to develop training for certain RME, but VA lacks a timeline for developing this training.

GAO also found weaknesses in VA's oversight of VAMCs' compliance with the selected purchasing and reprocessing requirements. These weaknesses render VA unable to systematically identify and address noncompliance with the requirements, which poses potential risks to the safety of veterans. GAO did not identify weaknesses in VA's oversight of VAMCs' compliance with the selected tracking requirements. GAO found the following:

- Oversight over purchasing requirements. In general, VA does not oversee VAMCs' compliance with the selected purchasing requirements. While VA intends to improve oversight over these requirements, it has not yet developed a plan for doing so.
- Oversight over reprocessing requirements. Although VA headquarters receives information from the VISNs on any noncompliance they identify as well as VAMCs' corrective action plans to address this noncompliance, VA headquarters does not analyze this information to inform its oversight. According to VA headquarters officials, VA intends to develop a plan for analyzing this information to systematically identify areas of noncompliance that occur frequently,

pose high risks to veterans' safety, or have not been addressed across all VAMCs.

May 3, 2011

The Honorable Jeff Miller
Chairman

The Honorable Bob Filner
Ranking Member
Committee on Veterans' Affairs
House of Representatives

The Honorable Charles E. Grassley
United States Senate

The Honorable Russ Carnahan
House of Representatives

The Department of Veterans Affairs (VA) operates one of the largest integrated health care delivery systems in the United States, providing care to over 5.5 million veterans annually. Organized into 21 Veterans Integrated Service Networks (VISN), VA's health care system includes 153 VA medical centers (VAMC) nationwide that offer a variety of outpatient, residential, and inpatient services.[1] In providing health care services to veterans, clinicians at VAMCs use supplies and equipment purchased by VA. These include expendable medical supplies, such as needles and scalpel blades, which are generally used once and discarded, and reusable medical equipment (RME), which is designed to be reused for multiple patients and includes such equipment as endoscopes and some surgical instruments. Because RME is used when providing care to multiple veterans, this equipment must be reprocessed—that is, cleaned and disinfected or sterilized—between uses. VA has established requirements for VAMCs to follow for purchasing items such as expendable medical supplies and RME; for tracking—that is, accounting for—these items at their facilities;[2] and for reprocessing RME.[3] These policies are designed, in part, to help ensure the safety of the veterans who receive care at VAMCs.

Recent press articles have reported lapses in compliance with VA's reprocessing requirements at some VA medical centers, which may have put the safety of thousands of veterans receiving care at these facilities at risk.[4] For example, one article reported that between 2009 and 2010, about 1,800 veterans were potentially exposed to infectious diseases at the St. Louis VAMC, because they received care using improperly reprocessed dental instruments.[5] Moreover, in a September 2010 congressional hearing, we presented our preliminary observations on veterans' safety issues related to expendable medical supplies and RME. We reported examples of noncompliance with VA's requirements for purchasing and tracking certain medical supplies and equipment, which may pose risks to veterans' safety. In response, a congressional committee and certain members of Congress have raised questions about the adequacy of VA's requirements for purchasing, tracking, and reprocessing to help ensure veterans' safety. In addition, questions have been raised regarding the adequacy of VA's oversight of VAMCs' compliance with these requirements. In this report, we examine (1) VA purchasing, tracking, and reprocessing requirements in VA policies, which were selected based on their relevance to patient safety incidents, and (2) VA's oversight of VAMCs' compliance with these selected requirements.

To examine VA purchasing, tracking, and reprocessing requirements, we reviewed relevant VA policies, and from these policies we judgmentally selected two purchasing requirements, two tracking requirements, and two reprocessing requirements that we determined were relevant to patient safety incidents that were identified at certain VAMCs.[6] After selecting these requirements for our review, we judgmentally selected six VAMCs from the following locations to visit: Albany, New York; Cheyenne, Wyoming; Detroit, Michigan; Miami, Florida; Palo Alto, California; and St. Louis, Missouri. These VAMCs represent different surgical complexity groups[7] and geographic regions[8] and serve veteran populations of different sizes. At these six VAMCs, we examined the adequacy of the selected purchasing, tracking, and reprocessing requirements to help the facilities ensure the safety of veterans who received care at these facilities. To do this, we examined how the selected requirements in these policies were implemented and whether or to what extent the selected requirements directly or indirectly created a potential risk to the safety of the veterans receiving care at the VAMCs. We reviewed applicable VAMC committee meeting minutes[9] and other documentation on the implementation of these requirements. We also interviewed VAMC officials who were responsible for implementing the selected requirements in VA policies to determine whether the selected requirements are adequate to help ensure veterans' safety.

To examine VA's oversight of VAMCs' compliance with the purchasing, tracking, and reprocessing requirements we selected, we reviewed VA's oversight of these requirements and evaluated whether this oversight provides VA with adequate information to identify and address noncompliance. As part of this review, we assessed VA's oversight in the context of federal standards for internal control for monitoring.[10] The internal control for monitoring refers to an agency's ability to assure that ongoing review and supervision activities are conducted, with the scope and frequency depending on the assessment of risks; deficiencies are communicated to at least one higher level of management; and actions are taken in response to findings or recommendations within established timelines. We interviewed officials responsible for overseeing VAMCs' compliance with the requirements we selected for review from VA headquarters, VA's Office of Inspector General (OIG), and six VISNs that are responsible for overseeing compliance at the VAMCs we visited. In addition, we obtained and reviewed relevant documents regarding VA oversight, including internal reports, VAMCs' plans to correct problems identified through oversight activities, and policy memorandums.

We conducted this performance audit from March 2010 to May 2011 in accordance with generally accepted government auditing standards. Those standards require that we plan and perform the audit to obtain sufficient, appropriate evidence to provide a reasonable basis for our findings and conclusions based on our audit objectives. We believe that the evidence obtained provides a reasonable basis for our findings and conclusions based on our audit objectives. See appendix I for more information on our scope and methodology.

BACKGROUND

VA is required by law to provide hospital care and medical services to certain veterans and may provide care to other veterans.[11] In general, veterans must enroll in VA health care to receive VA's medical benefits package that includes a range of services such as preventative health care services and inpatient hospital services. Veterans may receive certain other health care services, such as dental care, without enrolling.12 VA provides these services at various types of facilities, including VAMCs. In providing these services to veterans, clinicians at VAMCs use expendable medical supplies and RME. VA has established roles and responsibilities within its system for purchasing, tracking, and reprocessing of these items and policies that VAMCs are required to follow when purchasing and tracking these items at their facilities. VA also has policies that VAMCs are required to follow regarding the reprocessing of RME.

VA Roles and Responsibilities for Purchasing, Tracking, and Reprocessing

VA headquarters is responsible for the development of policies related to purchasing, tracking, and reprocessing and is ultimately responsible for ensuring that VISNs and VAMCs are in compliance with these policies. Within VA headquarters, the Office of Acquisition, Logistics, and Construction and the Procurement and Logistics Office, are responsible for policies related to the purchasing and tracking of expendable medical supplies and RME, while the Sterile Processing Department is responsible for policies related to the reprocessing of RME.

Each of the 21 regional VISNs is responsible for ensuring compliance with VA's policies at the VAMCs within its region. VISNs report to the Deputy Under Secretary for Health for Operations and Management within VA headquarters.

In turn, each of the 153 VAMCs is responsible for implementing VA's policies. Within each VAMC, the Acquisition Department is responsible for purchasing expendable medical supplies and RME, the Logistics Department is responsible for tracking these items, and the Sterile Processing Department is responsible for reprocessing RME. (See fig. 1 for an overview of VA's organizational structure.)

VA Policies for Purchasing, Tracking, and Reprocessing

VA policies specify how VAMCs can purchase expendable medical supplies and RME. VAMCs can purchase expendable medical supplies and RME through their acquisition departments or through their clinical departments, such as the radiology department. VA's policies include the following requirements related to veterans' safety that VAMCs must follow when purchasing expendable medical supplies and RME:

Committee review and approval. A designated VAMC committee must review and approve proposed purchases of any expendable medical supplies or RME that have not been previously purchased by the VAMC.[13]

The committee, which typically includes administrative staff and clinicians from various departments, reviews the proposed purchases to evaluate the cost of the purchase as well as its likely effect on veterans' care.[14] For example, the committee that reviews and approves proposed RME purchases often includes a representative from the department responsible for reprocessing RME in order to determine whether the VAMC has the capability to reprocess the item correctly and to ensure that staff are appropriately trained to do so.

Proper reprocessing of RME is important to ensure that RME is safe to use and that veterans are not exposed to infectious diseases, such as Human Immunodeficiency Virus (HIV), during treatment.

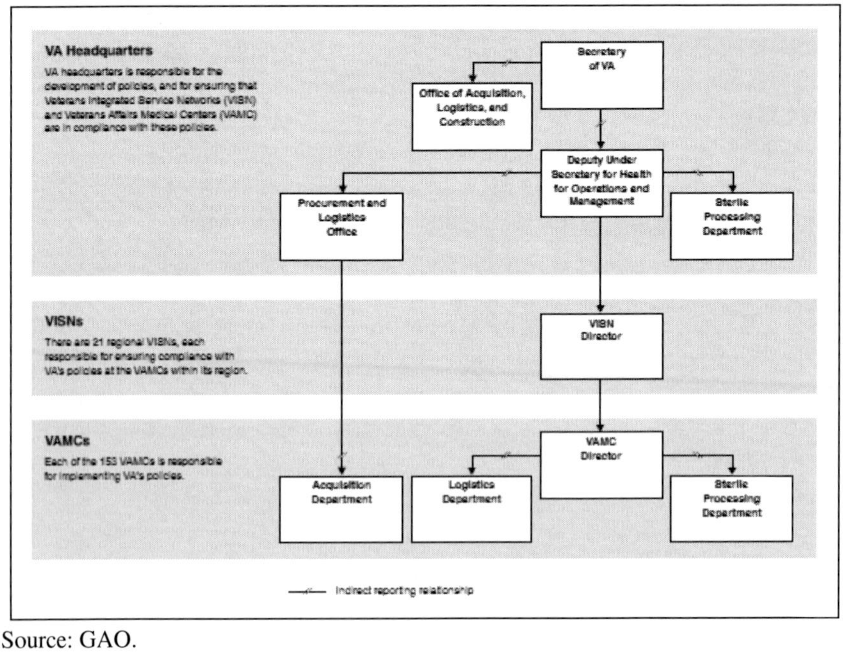

Source: GAO.

Figure 1. Selected Veterans Affairs (VA) Entities' Roles and Responsibilities for Purchasing, Tracking, and Reprocessing.

Signatures from two officials. All approvals for purchases of expendable medical supplies and RME must be signed by two officials, the official placing the order and the official responsible for approving the purchase.[15] This process helps ensure that purchases of expendable medical supplies and RME are appropriate to use when providing care to veterans.

VA has two inventory management systems that it requires VAMCs to use to track the type and quantity of expendable medical supplies and RME used in its facilities.

VAMCs use information about the items in their facilities for a variety of purposes, for example to readily determine whether they have expendable medical supplies or RME that are the subject of a manufacturer recall or a patient safety alert.

VA policy requires that each VAMC enter information about certain expendable medical supplies and RME in their facilities into the appropriate system.

Specifically, VA policies include two key requirements related to veterans' safety that VAMCs must follow for tracking expendable medical supplies and RME:

Tracking of expendable medical supplies. VAMCs must enter information on all expendable medical supplies that are ordered on a recurring basis into the Generic Inventory Package (GIP).[16]

Tracking of RME. VAMCs must enter information on all RME that is classified as nonexpendable equipment by VA's Office of Acquisition, Logistics, and Construction into the Automated Engineering Management System / Medical Equipment Reporting System (AEMS/MERS).[17]

VA policies include requirements designed to help ensure that VAMCs reprocess RME correctly,[18] in order to help ensure that RME is safe for use when providing care to veterans. VA's reprocessing policies include two key types of requirements:

Training requirements. To ensure that RME is reprocessed in accordance with manufacturers' guidelines, VA requires that each VAMC develop device-specific training for reprocessing RME.

To develop this training, VA requires VAMCs to create device-specific standard operating procedures (SOP), which provide step-by-step instructions for reprocessing.

VA also requires VAMCs to assess staff annually on their competence to reprocess RME in accordance with these SOPs.

Operational requirements. To ensure that reprocessing activities are performed safely and that RME is reprocessed correctly, VA policies establish operational requirements for VAMCs, which include that VAMC staff must monitor sterilizers to ensure that they are functioning properly, use personal protective equipment when performing reprocessing activities, and segregate dirty and clean RME.

Selected VA Requirements for Tracking and Reprocessing Are Inadequate to Help Ensure Veterans' Safety

We found that both the tracking and reprocessing requirements we reviewed are inadequate to help ensure the safety of veterans who receive care at VAMCs. These inadequacies create potential risks to the safety of veterans who receive care at VAMCs. However, we did not identify any inadequacies in the purchasing requirements we selected for review that may create potential risks to veterans' safety.

VAMCs Are Not Required to Track Certain Expendable Medical Supplies and RME

VA does not require VAMCs to enter information about certain expendable medical supplies and RME into their inventory management systems, and therefore, VAMC inventories have incomplete information on these items. Specifically, VAMCs are not required to enter into GIP information on expendable medical supplies purchased on a nonrecurring basis. Furthermore, VAMCs are not required to enter into AEMS/MERS information on RME that VA's Office of Acquisition, Logistics, and Construction does not classify as nonexpendable equipment. RME that is not classified as nonexpendable equipment includes certain surgical and dental instruments. As a result, none of the six VAMCs we visited had complete inventories of all of the expendable medical supplies or RME in their facilities. Incomplete inventories of these items at VAMCs can pose potential risks to veterans' safety.

At all six of the VAMCs we visited, we identified examples of potential risks to veterans' safety that may result from these inadequacies in VA's tracking requirements. For example:

Limited ability to identify items on which there are alerts or recalls. In the event of a manufacturer recall or patient safety alert related to an expendable medical supply item or RME, VAMCs may be unable to use their inventory management systems to systematically determine whether the affected item is in their facilities and should therefore be removed so that it is not used when providing care to veterans. Rather, VAMC officials would have to rely on a physical search for the item throughout their facilities—and a physical search could miss items. As we reported in our 2010 testimony,[19] VAMC officials and officials from the VA OIG told us that in response to a patient safety alert in December 2008 regarding an auxiliary water tube—a type of RME that is used with a colonoscope— VAMC officials checked their inventory management systems and concluded—incorrectly—that the tube was not used in the facility.[20] However, in March 2009, the VAMC discovered that the tube was in use in the facility and was not being reprocessed correctly, potentially exposing 2,526 veterans to infectious diseases such as HIV, hepatitis B, and hepatitis C.[21]

Difficulty maintaining appropriate inventories. Because GIP helps VAMCs to ensure that they maintain appropriate quantities of supply items in their facilities, VAMCs with incomplete information in GIP about the supplies in their facilities may have difficulty ensuring that they maintain appropriate quantities of these items. This may result in expendable medical supplies being unavailable for veterans' care if needed or, alternatively, excess supplies accumulating and expiring before they can be used. For example, in 2009 and 2010, VA headquarters officials identified expired expendable medical supplies, which were not being properly tracked in GIP, at three of the six VAMCs we visited. Had these VAMCs been properly tracking these supply items in GIP, they may have been able to maintain appropriate quantities of items and therefore avoid unavailable or expired supplies.

Challenges developing required training. VAMCs with incomplete information about the RME in their inventories face challenges identifying the equipment for which they must develop device-specific reprocessing training. None of the six VAMCs we visited relied on their inventory management systems to systematically determine which types of RME they had in their facilities. In fact, officials at all six VAMCs told us that they had to use alternate methods, such as contacting individual staff members or conducting searches in each clinical department, to determine if the facility had a specific type of RME. These methods of searching for RME make it difficult for VAMCs to ensure that they identify all of the RME in their facilities for which they must develop device-specific reprocessing training—without inadvertently missing items—and may have contributed to delays in developing this training. Approximately 1 year after VA instituted the requirement for developing device-specific training for reprocessing, three of the six VAMCs we visited had not yet fully developed this training. Without appropriate training for reprocessing RME, VAMCs cannot ensure that staff in their facilities are reprocessing RME correctly so that these items are safe for use when caring for veterans.

At the time of our review, VA did not have plans to immediately address the inadequacies we identified in the tracking requirements by requiring VAMCs to enter information about all expendable medical supplies and RME into VA's inventory management systems. VA headquarters officials told us that they plan to address the inadequacies we identified in the tracking requirements following implementation of a new inventory management system—Strategic Asset Management. However, VA had suspended the implementation of this system as of March 2011. Although VA did not plan on revising its tracking requirements immediately, officials from two of the six VAMCs we visited told us that they have taken steps to improve the information they maintain on the expendable medical supplies at their facilities. Officials told us that they are requiring staff to enter information about all expendable medical supplies at these VAMCs into GIP, including those that are purchased on a nonrecurring basis.

Selected VA Reprocessing Requirements Are Inadequate

The VA reprocessing requirements we selected for review are inadequate to help ensure veterans' safety in two respects: (1) they do not specify the types of RME for which VAMCs must develop device-specific training, and (2) VA has provided VAMCs with conflicting guidance on how to develop this training.[22]

Lack of specificity about types of RME that require device-specific training. The VA reprocessing requirements we reviewed do not specify the types of RME for which VAMCs must develop device-specific training. This inadequacy has caused confusion among VAMCs and contributed to inconsistent implementation of training for RME reprocessing. While VA headquarters officials told us that the training requirement is intended to apply to RME classified as critical—such as surgical instruments—and semi-critical—such as certain endoscopes,[23] officials from five of the six VAMCs we visited told us that they were unclear about the RME for which they were required to develop device-specific training.

Officials at one VAMC we visited told us that they did not develop all of the required reprocessing training for critical RME—such as surgical instruments—because they did not understand that they were required to do so. Officials at another VAMC we visited also told us that they had begun to develop device-specific training for reprocessing non-critical RME, such as wheelchairs, even though they had not yet fully completed device-specific training for more critical RME. Because these two VAMCs had not developed the appropriate device-specific training for reprocessing critical and semi-critical RME, staff at these VAMCs may not have been reprocessing all RME properly, which potentially put the safety of veterans receiving care at these facilities at risk.

Conflicting guidance on the development of RME reprocessing training. While VA requires VAMCs to develop device-specific training on reprocessing RME, VA headquarters officials provided VAMCs with conflicting guidance on how they should develop this training. For example, officials at three VAMCs we visited told us that certain VA headquarters or VISN officials stated that this device-specific training should very closely match manufacturer guidelines--in one case verbatim—while other VA headquarters or VISN officials stated that this training should be written in a way that could be easily understood by the personnel responsible for reprocessing the RME. This distinction is important, since VAMC officials told us that some of the staff responsible for reprocessing the RME may have difficulty following the more technical manufacturers' guidelines.[24] In part because of VA's conflicting guidance, VAMC officials told us that they had difficulty developing the required device-specific training and had to rewrite the training materials multiple times for RME at their facilities. Officials at five of the six VAMCs also told us that developing the device-specific training for reprocessing RME was both time consuming and resource intensive.

VA's lack of specificity and conflicting guidance regarding its requirement to develop device-specific training for reprocessing RME may have contributed to delays in developing this training at several of the VAMCs we visited. Officials from three of the six VAMCs told us that they had not completed the development of device-specific training for RME since VA established the training requirement in July 2009. As of October 2010, 15 months after VA issued the policy containing this requirement, officials at one of the VAMCs we visited told us that device-specific training on reprocessing had not been developed for about 80 percent of the critical and semi-critical RME in use at the facility.

VA headquarters officials told us that they are aware of the lack of specificity and conflicting guidance provided to VAMCs regarding the development of training for reprocessing RME, and were also aware of inefficiencies resulting from each VAMC developing its own training for reprocessing types of RME that are used in multiple VAMCs. In response, VA headquarters officials told us that they have made available to all VAMCS a database of standardized device-specific training developed by RME manufacturers for approximately 1,000 types of RME and plan to require VAMCs to implement this training by June 2011. The officials also told us that VA headquarters is planning to develop device-specific training available to all VAMCs for certain critical and semi-critical RME for which RME manufacturers have not developed this training, such as dental instruments. However, as of February 2011, VA headquarters has not completed device-specific training for these RME and has not established plans or corresponding timelines for completing this training.

VA's Oversight of VAMCs' Compliance with Selected Purchasing and Reprocessing Requirements Has Weaknesses

VA's oversight of VAMCs' compliance with selected purchasing and reprocessing requirements has weaknesses, which result in VA not being able to systematically identify and address noncompliance. We did not identify any weaknesses in VA's oversight of the tracking requirements we selected for review.[25] Oversight of VAMCs' compliance with the selected purchasing, tracking, and reprocessing requirements is important because, at each of the six VAMCs we visited, we identified examples of noncompliance, which may result in risks to veterans' safety. VA headquarters officials told us that VA intends to improve oversight over the selected purchasing requirements, but has not yet developed a plan for doing so. In addition, VA recently made changes to its oversight of VAMCs' compliance with selected reprocessing requirements; however, this oversight continues to have weaknesses.

VA Has Limited Oversight of VAMCs' Compliance with Selected Purchasing Requirements

We found that, in general, VA does not oversee VAMCs' compliance with the purchasing requirements we selected for review. Specifically, neither VA headquarters nor the six VISNs that oversee the VAMCs we visited provided oversight for the committee review and approval requirement and only one of the six VISNs provided oversight of the double signature requirement.[26] Consistent with the federal internal control for monitoring, which is applicable to all federal agencies, we would expect VA to oversee VAMCs' compliance with the requirements we selected, assess the risk of VAMCs' noncompliance with these requirements, and ensure that noncompliance is addressed.[27]

Without oversight of the selected purchasing requirements, VA is unable to identify and address VAMCs' noncompliance with the selected purchasing requirements. During our site visits to six VAMCs, we identified examples of noncompliance with these requirements that created potential risks to veterans' safety.[28] *VAMC committee review and approval.* Officials from four of the six VAMCs we visited told us that certain expendable medical supplies—for example, those used in a limited number of clinical departments—were sometimes purchased without the required VAMC committee review and approval. Furthermore, officials from one of those four VAMCs told us that none of the expendable medical supplies it purchased were reviewed and approved by a VAMC committee. Without obtaining the required review and approval, these VAMCs may have purchased expendable medical supplies without evaluating their cost-effectiveness or likely effect on veterans' care.

Signatures of purchasing and approving officials. At one of the six VAMCs we visited, VAMC officials discovered that one staff member working in a dialysis department purchased expendable medical supplies without obtaining the required signature of an appropriate approving official. That staff member ordered the wrong supplies, which incorrectly allowed blood to pass into dialysis machines. Those supplies were used for 83 veterans, resulting in potential cross-contamination of these veterans' blood, which may have exposed them to infectious diseases, such as HIV, hepatitis B, and hepatitis C.[29] In January 2011, VA headquarters officials told us that they intend to develop an approach to oversee VAMCs' compliance with the selected purchasing requirements, although VA has not yet established a timeline for developing and implementing this oversight. In addition, an official from one VISN told us in January 2011 that the VISN planned to begin overseeing VAMCs' compliance with VA's requirement that two signatures be obtained for purchases of expendable medical supplies and RME. However, the official told us that the VISN had not yet established a timeline for developing and implementing this oversight.

Despite Changes Intended to Improve Its Oversight of VAMCs' Compliance with Selected Reprocessing Requirements, VA's Oversight Has Weaknesses

Beginning in fiscal year 2011, VA headquarters directed VISNs to make three changes intended to improve its oversight of VAMCs' compliance with the selected reprocessing requirements at VAMCs.[30]

- VA headquarters recently required VISNs to increase the frequency of site visits to VAMCs—from one to three unannounced site visits per year—as a way to more quickly identify and address areas of noncompliance with selected VA reprocessing requirements.
- VA headquarters also recently required VISNs to begin using a standardized assessment tool to guide their oversight activities.[31] According to VA headquarters officials, requiring VISNs to use this assessment tool will enable the VISNs to collect consistent information on VAMCs' compliance with VA's reprocessing requirements. Before VA established this requirement, the six VISNs that oversee the VAMCs we visited often used different assessment tools to guide their oversight activities. As a result, they reviewed and collected different types of information on VAMCs' compliance with these requirements.
- VISNs are now required to report to VA headquarters information from their site visits. Specifically, following each unannounced site visit to each VAMC, VISNs are required to provide VA headquarters with information on VAMCs' noncompliance with VA's reprocessing requirements and VAMCs' corrective action plans to address areas of noncompliance. Prior to fiscal year 2011, VISNs were generally not required to report this information to VA headquarters.[32]

Despite the recent changes, VA's oversight of VAMCs' compliance with its reprocessing requirements, including those we selected for review, has weaknesses in the context of the federal internal control for monitoring. Consistent with the internal control for monitoring, we would expect VA to analyze this information to assess the risk of noncompliance and ensure that noncompliance is addressed. However, VA headquarters does not analyze information to identify the extent of noncompliance across all VAMCs, including noncompliance that occurs frequently or poses high risks to veterans' safety. As a result, VA headquarters has not identified the extent of noncompliance across all VAMCs with, for example, VA's operational reprocessing requirement that staff use personal protective equipment when performing reprocessing activities, which is key to ensuring that clean RME are not contaminated by coming into contact with soiled hands or clothing. Three of the six VAMCs we visited had instances of noncompliance with this requirement. Similarly, because VA headquarters does not analyze information from VAMCs' corrective action plans to address noncompliance with VA reprocessing requirements, it is unable to confirm, for example, whether

VAMCs have addressed noncompliance with its operational reprocessing requirement to separate clean and dirty RME. Two of the six VAMCs we visited had not resolved noncompliance with this requirement. Compliance with this requirement is important to ensure that clean RME does not become contaminated by coming into contact with dirty RME.

VA headquarters officials told us that VA plans to address the weaknesses we identified in its oversight of VAMCs' compliance with reprocessing requirements. Specifically, VA headquarters officials told us that they intend to develop a systematic approach to analyze the information on VAMCs' noncompliance and corrective action plans to identify areas of noncompliance across all VAMCs, including those that occur frequently, pose high risks to veterans' safety, or have not been addressed in a timely manner.[33] While VA has established a timeline for completing these changes, certain VA headquarters officials told us that they are unsure whether this timeline is realistic due to possible delays resulting from VA's ongoing organizational realignment, which had not been completed as of April 6, 2011.[34]

CONCLUSION

Weaknesses exist in VA's processes for tracking expendable medical supplies and RME and reprocessing RME that create potential safety risks to veterans. Because VA does not require VAMCs to track information about certain expendable medical supplies and RME in their inventory management systems, VAMCs may be unaware of the complete inventory of such items at their facilities. This knowledge is critical to maintain available supplies on hand to serve veterans, to properly identify items for which manufacturers have issued recalls, and to develop training on reprocessing the RME in their inventory. Moreover, VA's lack of specificity and conflicting guidance for developing device-specific training for reprocessing RME has led to confusion among VAMCs about which types of RME require device-specific training and how VAMCs should develop that training. This confusion has contributed to some VAMCs not developing training for their staff for some critical and semi-critical RME. Until these weaknesses are addressed, the safety of veterans receiving care at VAMCs could potentially be at risk.

A general lack of oversight of VAMCs' compliance with selected purchasing requirements makes it difficult for VA to identify and resolve situations wherein items are purchased without proper review and approval. A failure to review and approve these purchases poses safety risks to veterans being treated in VAMCs. In fact, during our visits to VAMCs, we noted examples of expendable medical supplies that were purchased without appropriate review and approval.

As a result, some supplies may have been purchased without evaluating the likely effect on veterans' care, or worse yet, the wrong supplies were ordered—a mistake that potentially led to some veterans being exposed to infectious diseases. Furthermore, weaknesses in oversight of VAMCs' compliance with the selected reprocessing requirements do not allow VA to identify and subsequently address areas of noncompliance across all VAMCs, including those that occur frequently, pose high risks to veterans' safety, or have not been addressed by VAMCs. Providing effective oversight over purchasing and reprocessing requirements consistent with the federal standards for internal control would help VA prevent potentially harmful incidents from occurring.

RECOMMENDATIONS FOR EXECUTIVE ACTION

To help ensure veterans' safety through VA's purchasing, tracking, and reprocessing requirements, we are making four recommendations. We recommend that the Secretary of Veterans Affairs direct the Under Secretary for Health to take the following four actions:

- Require VAMCs to enter information about all expendable medical supplies and RME into an appropriate inventory management system.
- Develop and implement an approach for providing standardized training for reprocessing all critical and semi-critical RME to VAMCs. Additionally, hold VAMCs accountable for implementing device-specific training for all of these RME.
- Develop and implement an approach to oversee compliance at all VAMCs with the selected purchasing requirements.
- Use the information on noncompliance identified by the VISNs and information on VAMCs' corrective action plans to identify areas of noncompliance across all 153 VAMCs, including those that occur frequently, pose high risks to veterans' safety, or have not been addressed, and take action to improve compliance in those areas.

Agency Comments and Our Evaluation

VA provided written comments on a draft of this report. In its comments, VA concurred with our recommendations and described the department's planned actions to implement them. VA also provided technical comments, which we incorporated, as appropriate.

To address our recommendation that VA require VAMCs to enter information about all expendable medical supplies and RME into an appropriate inventory management system, VA stated that it plans to take several actions that include the following. By September 30, 2011, the department plans to implement a process for tracking information on certain expendable medical supplies, which are currently not being tracked in GIP, to ensure that these items can be identified in the event of a recall. Furthermore, by September 30, 2011, VA plans to implement a pilot program for tracking certain RME, such as surgical and dental instruments, which are currently not being tracked in AEMS/MERS.

To address our recommendation that VA develop an approach for providing standardized training to VAMCs on reprocessing all critical and semi-critical RME, VA stated that it is taking several actions, which include revising VA's requirement for developing device-specific reprocessing training and providing staff training through a professional organization that specializes in RME reprocessing. In our report, we stated that VA headquarters is planning to develop device-specific training available to all VAMCs for certain critical and semi-critical RME for which RME manufacturers have not developed this training, such as dental instruments, but had not developed a time frame for developing this training. VA's comments did not provide an update on when this training would be developed. To hold VAMCs accountable for implementing training for critical and semi-critical RME, VA reiterated that it is strengthening its oversight of VAMCs and is requiring VAMCs to develop corrective action plans to ensure that noncompliance with the training requirement is addressed.

To address our recommendation that VA develop and implement an approach to oversee compliance with selected purchasing requirements at all VAMCs, VA stated that it plans to oversee VAMCs' purchasing activities, including VAMCs' compliance with our selected purchasing requirements. To do this, VA stated that by September 30, 2011, VA headquarters' Purchasing and Logistics Office will begin requiring VISN officials to conduct routine site visits to VAMCs to help the latter develop action plans for addressing noncompliance with the purchasing requirements. The Purchasing and

Logistics Office also plans to review and approve these action plans and follow up with VAMCs to ensure that any noncompliance is addressed.

To address our recommendation that VA use information on noncompliance to identify areas of noncompliance across all VAMCs and take action to improve compliance in those areas, VA plans to analyze the results of its oversight activities to identify national concerns and target future Sterile Processing Department initiatives. In our report we stated that while VA has established a timeline for conducting this analysis, certain VA headquarters officials told us that they were unsure whether this timeline is realistic. In its comments, VA did not provide information on whether it anticipates meeting its expected timeline. VA also reiterated changes that it has made that are intended to improve its oversight of VAMCs' compliance with its requirements.

Randall B. Williamson
Director, Health Care

APPENDIX I: SCOPE AND METHODOLOGY

To examine Department of Veterans Affairs (VA) purchasing, tracking, and reprocessing requirements, we reviewed relevant VA policies[1] and from these policies we judgmentally selected two purchasing requirements, two tracking requirements, and two reprocessing requirements that we determined were relevant to veterans' safety issues that were identified at certain VA medical centers (VAMC) in 2008 and 2009. Specifically, the purchasing requirements we selected were relevant to a patient safety incident at the VAMC in Palo Alto, California, resulting from the improper purchase and use of dialysis supplies; the tracking requirements we selected were relevant to a patient safety incident resulting from the improper reprocessing of endoscopy equipment at the VAMC in Miami, Florida; and the reprocessing requirements we selected were relevant to patient safety incidents resulting from the improper reprocessing of endoscopy equipment at the VAMCs in Augusta, Georgia; Miami, Florida; and Murfreesboro, Tennessee.

After selecting these requirements for our review, we judgmentally selected six VAMCs at the following locations to visit: Albany, New York; Cheyenne, Wyoming; Detroit, Michigan; Miami, Florida; Palo Alto, California; and St. Louis, Missouri. These VAMCs represent different surgical complexity groups,[2] serve veteran populations of different sizes, and are located in different Veterans Integrated Service Networks (VISN). (See table 1.)

Table 1. Characteristics of VAMCs Selected for Site Visits

VAMC location	Surgical complexity group[a]	Size of patient population served, 2009	VISN
Albany, New York	2	Greater than 24,999 and less than 50,000	2
Cheyenne, Wyoming	3	Less than 25,000	19
Detroit, Michigan	1[c]	Greater than 24,999 and less than 50,000	11
Miami, Florida	1[b]	Greater than 49,999	8
Palo Alto, California	1[a]	Greater than 49,999	21
St. Louis, Missouri	1[a]	Greater than 49,999	15

Source: GAO analysis of VA data.

[a] A assigns each VAMC a complexity score between 1 and 3, with level 1 being the most complex, using a facility complexity model. Level 1 is broken down further into 1a, 1b, and 1c. That model uses multiple variables to measure facility complexity arrayed along four categories, namely patient population served, clinical services offered, education and research complexity, and administrative complexity.

At these six VAMCs, we examined the adequacy of the selected purchasing, tracking, and reprocessing requirements to help ensure the safety of veterans who received care. To do this, we examined how the requirements in these policies were implemented and whether the requirements indirectly created a potential risk to the safety of veterans who receive care at VAMCs. Specifically, at each VAMC we visited, we reviewed applicable VAMC committee meeting minutes[3] and other documentation on the implementation of these requirements. We also interviewed VAMC officials who were responsible for implementing the selected requirements to determine whether the requirements were adequate to help ensure veterans' safety. At each VAMC, these officials included members of the executive leadership team, the nurse executive, the chief of the Sterile Processing Department, the patient safety manager, infection preventionists, and members of the quality management staff.[4]

To examine VA's oversight of VAMCs' compliance with the purchasing, tracking, and reprocessing requirements we selected, we reviewed VA's oversight of these requirements and evaluated whether this oversight provides VA with adequate information to identify and address noncompliance. As part of this review, we reviewed VA's oversight in the context of federal standards for internal control for monitoring.[5] The internal control for monitoring refers to an agency's ability to assure that ongoing review and supervision activities are conducted, with the scope and frequency depending on the assessment of risks, deficiencies are communicated to at least one higher level of management, and actions are taken in response to findings or recommendations within established timelines.

We then interviewed officials from VA headquarters, including the Sterile Processing Department, the Infectious Disease Program Office, and the System-wide Ongoing Assessment and Review Strategy; VA's Office of Inspector General; and the six VISNs that oversee the VAMCs we visited who are responsible for overseeing compliance with VA's requirements, including those we selected for our review. Through our interviews, we obtained information on the oversight activities conducted by each of these entities and the extent to which these entities followed up with VAMCs to ensure that they corrected problems identified through these oversight activities. In addition, we obtained and reviewed relevant documents regarding VA oversight, including internal reports, VAMCs' plans to correct problems identified through oversight activities, and policy memorandums.

We conducted this performance audit from March 2010 to May 2011 in accordance with generally accepted government auditing standards. Those standards require that we plan and perform the audit to obtain sufficient, appropriate evidence to provide a reasonable basis for our findings and conclusions based on our audit objectives. We believe that the evidence obtained provides a reasonable basis for our findings and conclusions based on our audit objectives.

End Notes

[1] The management of VAMCs is decentralized to 21 VISNs.

[2] See, for example, VA Handbook 7176, Supply, Processing, and Distribution (SPD) Operational Requirements (Aug. 16, 2002) and Veterans Health Administration (VHA) Handbook 1761.02, VHA Inventory Management (Oct. 20, 2009).

[3] VA Handbook 7176, Supply, Processing, and Distribution (SPD) Operational Requirements; VHA Directive 2009-004, Use and Reprocessing of Reusable Medical Equipment (RME) in Veterans Health Administration Facilities (Feb. 9, 2009); and VHA Directive 2009-031,

Improving Safety in the Use of Reusable Medical Equipment Through Standardization of Organizational Structure and Reprocessing Requirements (June 26, 2009).

4 According to press articles, patient safety incidents involving improperly reprocessed RME have also occurred at non-VA hospitals. For example, a Pittsburgh Tribune-Review article from September 16, 2009, noted that patients at a non-VA hospital in Pennsylvania were potentially exposed to infectious diseases due to the improper reprocessing of surgical instruments. See W.F. Roche, "UPMC's Venango County facility improperly sterilized equipment," TribLIVE News (Sept. 16, 2009). Accessed on February 16, 2011, at http://www.pittsburghlive.com/x/leadertimes/s_643419.html.

5 See M. Owens, "St. Louis VA Medical Center dental infections: Nearly 2,000 at risk," KSDK.com (June 29, 2010). Accessed on February 16, 2011, at http://www.ksdk.com/news/local/story.aspx?catid=3&storyid=205262.

6 We reviewed applicable VA policies, including VHA Handbook 1761.02, VHA Inventory Management; VHA Directive 2009-031, Improving Safety in the Use of Reusable Medical Equipment Through Standardization of Organizational Structure and Reprocessing Requirements; VHA Directive 2009-004, Use and Reprocessing of Reusable Medical Equipment (RME) in Veterans Health Administration Facilities; VA Handbook 7002, Logistics Management Procedures (July 10, 2009); VA Handbook 7176, Supply, Processing, and Distribution (SPD) Operational Requirements; and VA Standard Operating Procedure #AM 5, Inventory of Equipment in Use Standard Operating Procedure (Feb. 17, 2011).

7 VA assigns each VAMC a complexity score between 1 and 3, with level 1 being the most complex, using a facility complexity model. Level 1 is broken down further into 1a, 1b, and 1c. That model uses multiple variables to measure facility complexity arrayed along four categories, namely patient population served, clinical services offered, education and research complexity, and administrative complexity.

8 Each of the six VAMCs we visited is located within a different VISN.

9 We reviewed minutes from the following committees: commodity standards, equipment, medical executive, infection control, and RME.

10 See GAO, Standards for Internal Control in the Federal Government, GAO/AIMD-00-21.3.1 (Washington, D.C.: November 1999) and GAO, Internal Control Management and Evaluation Tool, GAO-01-1008G (Washington, D.C.: August 2001).

11 38 U.S.C. §§ 1710(a)(1)-(3), 1701(5), (6). Requirements for VA health care services are effective in any fiscal year only to the extent and in the amount provided in advance in appropriations acts for such purposes. 38 U.S.C. § 1710(a)(4).

12 See 38 C.F.R. § 17.37 (2010).

13 Generally, a VAMC's commodity standards committee reviews and approves purchases of expendable medical supplies and a VAMC's equipment committee reviews and approves purchases of RME.

14 See VA Handbook 7176, Supply, Processing, and Distribution (SPD) Operational Requirements.

15 VA Handbook 7002, Logistics Management Procedures.

16 According to VHA Handbook 1730.01, Use and Management of the Government Purchase Card Program (Aug. 27, 2008), purchases are defined as recurring if they are made four or more times per year. In contrast, VHA Handbook 1761.02, VHA Inventory Management, states that expendable medical supplies that are ordered on a recurring basis must be entered into GIP but does not specify the number of times per year a purchase must be made in order to qualify as recurring.

[17] Nonexpendable equipment has a life expectancy of 2 years or more. See VA Standard Operating Procedure #AM 5, Inventory of Equipment in Use Standard Operating Procedure and VA Handbook 7002, Logistics Management Procedures.

[18] See VA Handbook 7176, Supply, Processing, and Distribution (SPD) Operational Requirements, VHA Directive 2009-004, Use and Reprocessing of Reusable Medical Equipment (RME) in Veterans Health Administration Facilities, and VHA Directive 2009-031, Improving Safety in the Use of Reusable Medical Equipment Through Standardization of Organizational Structure and Reprocessing Requirements.

[19] See GAO, VA Health Care: Preliminary Observations on the Purchasing and Tracking of Supplies and Medical Equipment and the Potential Impact on Veterans' Safety, GAO-10-1038T (Washington, D.C.: Sept. 23, 2010).

[20] Officials from this VAMC also checked with staff responsible for reprocessing in the gastrointestinal department, which is where colonoscopies are performed, to determine whether the VAMC possessed this type of RME. See VA Office of Inspector General, Use and Reprocessing of Flexible Fiberoptic Endoscopes at VA Medical Facilities, 09-01784-146 (Washington, D.C.: June 2009).

[21] As of August 17, 2010, the VAMC reported that it has successfully notified 2,523 of the 2,526 veterans of possible exposure to infectious diseases and that there were 17 new positive test results. VA reports that these results are not necessarily linked to RME issues and it is continuing its evaluation.

[22] According to VA headquarters officials, certain RME are difficult to reprocess because they need to be fully disassembled in order to be reprocessed correctly, so developing device-specific training for reprocessing these items is important to help ensure veterans' safety.

[23] RME is generally categorized into critical, semi-critical, or non-critical items based on the degree of risk for infection involved in use of the item. Critical items, such as surgical instruments, are those that enter sterile tissue or the vascular system and require sterilization because they confer a high risk of infection. Semi-critical items, such as certain endoscopes, are those that contact mucous membranes or non-intact skin and minimally require high-level disinfection. Non-critical items, such as wheelchairs, are those that come into contact with intact skin and may be cleaned with low-level disinfectants.

[24] VA officials stated that manufacturer guidelines for reprocessing RME may be technically complex and may include steps that VAMCs are unable to follow. For example, these officials stated that guidelines from RME manufacturers may require the use of a specific disinfectant that is not available in the United States. The Food and Drug Administration has responsibility for overseeing RME, including the guidelines written by manufacturers for reprocessing these items.

[25] VA headquarters' Management Quality Assurance Service (MQAS) oversees each VAMC's compliance with the selected VA tracking requirements approximately once every 7 to 8 years as part of broader compliance reviews. MQAS uses a standardized checklist to conduct these reviews. Following each review, VAMCs are required to develop corrective action plans to address areas of noncompliance. MQAS subsequently analyzes information on VAMC noncompliance and corrective action plans to identify the extent of noncompliance across all VAMCs, including those that occur frequently or have not been resolved. Although we did not identify any weaknesses in VA's oversight of the selected tracking requirements, as described earlier in this report, we did identify inadequacies in those requirements that pose risks to the safety of veterans.

[26] VA policy requires VISNs to conduct annual audits of some purchases—those made using purchase cards—which may include examining whether the two required signatures were

obtained. However, according to a VA headquarters official, these audits are conducted inconsistently across VISNs. See VHA Handbook 1730.01, Use and Management of the Government Purchase Card Program.

27 The federal internal control for monitoring states that an agency should be able to ensure that ongoing review and supervision activities are conducted, with the scope and frequency depending on the assessment of risks, and that actions in response to findings or recommendations are taken within established timelines. See GAO/AIMD-00-21.3.1 and GAO-01-1008G.

28 We previously reported examples of noncompliance with selected VA purchasing and tracking requirements from five VAMCs we visited. See GAO-10-1038T. We have since conducted a site visit to a sixth VAMC.

29 As of June 2, 2010, the VAMC reported that all testing has been completed and that no veterans have acquired infectious diseases as a result of this incident. The VAMC found that 1 of the 83 veterans identified was dialyzed on an uncontaminated machine and therefore this veteran was not notified or tested for these infectious diseases.

30 VA headquarters generally delegates responsibility for this oversight to the VISNs. In addition to oversight conducted by the VISNs, some entities within VA headquarters conduct oversight of VAMCs' compliance with VA reprocessing requirements, including those we selected for review. Specifically, VA's OIG and Sterile Processing Department conduct site visits to investigate allegations of VAMC noncompliance with VA reprocessing requirements. In addition, since around 2005, the System-wide Ongoing Assessment and Review Strategy has included reviews of the selected VA reprocessing requirements as part of broader reviews of VAMC compliance with VA policies in preparation for external accreditation reviews approximately every 3 years. In 2010, VA's OIG also conducted reviews of the selected VA reprocessing requirements as part of broader ongoing reviews of VAMC compliance with VA policies.

31 VA headquarters officials told us that they may refine this assessment tool over time.

32 While VISNs were not generally required to report to VA headquarters information on VAMCs' noncompliance with VA's reprocessing requirements, VISNs were required to report to VA headquarters information about noncompliance that may have resulted in harm to veterans. VA headquarters officials told us that, following a review of that information and collection of additional information, as needed, a panel of experts would determine whether the noncompliance identified in the reviews resulted in risks to veterans' safety and, if so, whether veterans should be notified. See VHA Directive 2008- 002, Disclosure of Adverse Events to Patients (Washington, D.C.: Jan. 18, 2008).

33 VA headquarters officials also told us that a temporary staff member was assigned in March 2011 to begin reviewing some information from VISNs' oversight activities. Specifically, that staff member will be responsible for reviewing whether VAMCs have developed the required device-specific training for reprocessing RME and the extent to which VAMCs are utilizing flash sterilization, a sterilization technique that should be used only in limited circumstances.

34 As part of this realignment, VA headquarters is establishing a new position within the Office of the Deputy Under Secretary for Health for Operations and Management, which will be responsible for overseeing certain departments, including VA headquarters' Sterile Processing Department.

End Notes for Appendix I

[1] We reviewed applicable VA policies, including VHA Handbook 1761.02, VHA Inventory Management (Oct. 20, 2009); VHA Directive 2009-031, Improving Safety in the Use of Reusable Medical Equipment Through Standardization of Organizational Structure And Reprocessing Requirements (June 26, 2009); VHA Directive 2009-004, Use and Reprocessing of Reusable Medical Equipment (RME) in Veterans Health Administration Facilities (Feb. 9, 2009); VA Handbook 7002, Logistics Management Procedures (July 10, 2009); VA Handbook 7176, Supply, Processing and Distribution (SPD) Operational Requirements (Aug. 16, 2002); and VA Standard Operating Procedure #AM 5, Inventory of Equipment in Use Standard Operating Procedure (Feb. 17, 2011).

[2] VA assigns each VAMC a complexity score between 1 and 3, with level 1 being the most complex, using a facility complexity model. Level 1 is broken down further into 1a, 1b, and 1c. That model uses multiple variables to measure facility complexity arrayed along four categories, namely patient population served, clinical services offered, education and research complexity, and administrative complexity.

[3] We reviewed minutes from the following committees: commodity standards, equipment, medical executive, infection control, and reusable medical equipment (RME).

[4] The patient safety manager is responsible for overseeing the response to patient safety advisories and alerts from VA headquarters and for addressing patient safety incidents at the VAMC; infection preventionists are responsible for helping to ensure that infection control standards are followed by VAMC staff; and the quality management staff is responsible for monitoring the quality of care at VAMCs.

[5] See GAO, Standards for Internal Control in the Federal Government, GAO/AIMD-00-21.3.1 (Washington, D.C.: November 1999) and GAO, Internal Control Management and Evaluation Tool, GAO-01-1008G (Washington, D.C.: August 2001).

In: Veteran's Health Care
Editor: Claude Da Costa

ISBN: 978-1-62417-371-4

Chapter 6

VETERANS' MEDICAL CARE: FY2013 APPROPRIATIONS*

Sidath Viranga Panangala

SUMMARY

The Department of Veterans Affairs (VA) provides benefits to veterans who meet certain eligibility criteria. Benefits to veterans range from disability compensation and pensions to hospital and medical care. The VA provides these benefits through three major operating units: the Veterans Health Administration (VHA), the Veterans Benefits Administration (VBA), and the National Cemetery Administration (NCA).

This report focuses on the VHA. The VHA is primarily a direct service provider of primary care, specialized care, and related medical and social support services to veterans through the nation's largest integrated health care system. Veterans generally must enroll in the VA health care system to receive medical care. Eligibility for enrollment is based primarily on previous military service, disability, and income. VA provides free inpatient and outpatient medical care to veterans for service-connected conditions and to low-income veterans for nonservice-connected conditions. The President's budget request was submitted to Congress on February 13, 2012. The President's budget is requesting

* This is an edited, reformatted and augmented version of a Congressional Research Service publication, CRS Report for Congress R42518, from www.crs.gov, prepared for Members and Committees of Congress, dated June 18, 2012.

$135.6 billion in budget authority for the VA as a whole. This includes approximately $75 billion in mandatory funding and $61 billion in discretionary funding. For FY2013, the Administration requests $53.3 billion for VHA. This includes $41.5 billion for the medical services account, $5.7 billion for the medical support and compliance account, $5.4 billion for the medical facilities account, and nearly $583 million for the medical and prosthetic research account. The total request for VHA represents a 4.1% increase over the FY2012-enacted appropriations. Furthermore, as required by the Veterans Health Care Budget Reform and Transparency Act of 2009 (P.L. 111-81), the President's budget is requesting $54.2 billion in advance appropriations for the three medical care accounts (medical services, medical support and compliance, and medical facilities) for FY2014.

The Senate Appropriations Committee, Military Construction, Veterans Affairs Subcommittee approved its version of a draft Military Construction and Veterans Affairs and Related Agencies Appropriations bill for FY2013 (MILCON-VA Appropriations bill) on May 15, 2012; the full Senate Appropriations Committee reported the draft measure on May 22. The Senate Appropriations Committee-reported MILCON-VA Appropriations bill (S. 3215; S.Rept. 112-168) provides a total of $135.6 billion for VA and, within that amount, a total of $53.3 billion is for VHA for FY2013. The total amount for VHA is approximately $2.1 billion above the FY2012- enacted amount and $10 million less than the Administration's request.

On May 31, 2012, the House passed its version of the MILCON-VA Appropriations bill for FY2013. The MILCON-VA Appropriations bill for FY2013 (H.R. 5854; H.Rept. 112-491) provides a total of $135.4 billion for the VA and, within that amount, a total of $53.1 billion is for VHA for FY2013. The total amount for VHA is approximately $2.0 billion above the FY2012- enacted amount and 0.3% less than the Administration's budget request for FY2013. Furthermore, as required by the Veterans Health Care Budget Reform and Transparency Act of 2009 (P.L. 111- 81), the House-passed and Senate Appropriations Committee reported MILCON-VA Appropriations bills (H.R. 5854; S. 3215) provide $54.2 billion in advance appropriations for the three medical care accounts (medical services, medical support and compliance, and medical facilities) for FY2014.

INTRODUCTION

The Department of Veterans Affairs (VA) provides a range of benefits and services to veterans[1] who meet certain eligibility rules; these benefits include medical care, disability compensation and pensions,[2] education,[3] vocational rehabilitation and employment services,[4] assistance to homeless veterans,[5] home loan guarantees,[6] administration of life insurance as well as traumatic injury protection insurance for servicemembers,[7] and death benefits that cover burial expenses.[8]

The VA carries out its programs nationwide through three administrations and the Board of Veterans Appeals (BVA). The Veterans Benefits Administration (VBA) is responsible for, among other things, providing compensation, pensions, and education assistance. The National Cemetery Administration (NCA)[9] is responsible for maintaining national veterans' cemeteries; providing grants to states for establishing, expanding, or improving state veterans' cemeteries; and providing headstones and markers for the graves of eligible persons, among other things. The Veterans Health Administration (VHA) is responsible for health care services and medical and prosthetic research programs. The VHA is primarily a direct service provider of primary care, specialized care, and related medical and social support services to veterans through the nation's largest integrated health care system. The VHA is also a provider of health care education and training for physician residents and other health care trainees.

In general, eligibility for VA health care is based on veteran status,[10] presence of service-connected disabilities[11] or exposures,[12] income,[13] and/or other factors, such as status as a former prisoner of war or receipt of a Purple Heart. Veterans who served in a theater of combat operations after November 11, 1998, have a special five-year post-discharge period of eligibility, during which they may enroll without having to meet income requirements or demonstrate a service-connected disability.[14]

Veterans generally must enroll in the VA health care system to receive medical care. Once enrolled, veterans are assigned to one of eight categories (see *Table A-1*).[15] It should be noted that in any given year, not all enrolled veterans obtain their health care services from VA. While some veterans may rely solely on VA for their care, others may receive the majority of their health care services from other sources, such as Medicare, Medicaid, private health insurance, and the military health system (TRICARE).[16] VA-enrolled veterans do not pay premiums or enrollment fees to receive care from the VA; however, they may incur out-of-pocket costs for VA care related to conditions that are not service-connected.[17]

This report focuses on appropriations for VHA. It begins with a brief overview of the VA's budget for FY2012 (the current fiscal year) and the President's request for FY2013 as a whole. It then presents a brief overview of VHA's budget formulation, a description of the accounts that fund the VHA, and a summary of the FY2012 VHA budget. The report ends with a section discussing recent legislative developments pertaining to the FY2013 VHA budget.

Advance Appropriations[18]

In order to understand annual appropriations for the Veterans Health Administration (VHA), it is essential to briefly discuss the role of advance appropriations. In 2009, Congress enacted the Veterans Health Care Budget Reform and Transparency Act of 2009 (P.L. 111-81) authorizing advance appropriations for three of the four accounts that comprise VHA: medical services, medical support and compliance, and medical facilities. [19] The fourth account, the medical and prosthetic research account, is not funded as an advance appropriation. P.L. 111-81 also required the Department of Veterans Affairs to submit a request for advance appropriations for VHA with its budget request each year.

Congress first provided advance appropriations for the three VHA accounts in the FY2010 appropriations cycle. The Consolidated Appropriations Act, 2010 (P.L. 111-117), provided advance appropriations for FY2011; the Department of Defense and Full-Year Continuing Appropriations Act, 2011 (P.L. 112-10), provided advance appropriations for FY2012; and the Consolidated Appropriations Act, 2012 (P.L. 112-74), enacted into law on December 23, 2011, provided advance appropriations for FY2013.

Under current budget scoring guidelines, new budget authority for an advance appropriation is scored in the fiscal year in which the funds become available for obligation.

Therefore, throughout the funding tables of this report, advance appropriations numbers are shown under the label "memorandum" and in the corresponding fiscal year column.

For example, advance appropriations for FY2013 authorized by the Consolidated Appropriations Act, 2012 (P.L. 112- 74), are shown under a separate memorandum and in the FY2013 column. However, it should be noted that budget authority for FY2013 refers to the budget authority authorized in P.L. 112-74 and any additional funding provided by the Military Construction and Veterans Affairs and Related Agencies Appropriations bill for FY2013 (H.R. 5854, H.Rept. 112-491; S. 3215, S.Rept. 112-168) that includes funding for the medical and prosthetic research account (the account that is not funded as an advance appropriations).

DEPARTMENT OF VETERANS AFFAIRS BUDGET

The VA budget includes both mandatory[20] and discretionary funding.[21] Mandatory accounts fund disability compensation, pensions, vocational rehabilitation and employment, education, life insurance, housing, and burial benefits (such as graveliners, outer burial receptacles, and headstones), among other benefits and services. Discretionary accounts fund medical care, medical research, construction programs, information technology, and general operating expenses, among other things.

Figure 1 provides a breakdown of FY2012 (current fiscal year) budget allocations for both mandatory and discretionary programs. In FY2012, the total VA budget authority was approximately $122.2 billion; discretionary budget authority accounted for about 49% ($58.5 billion) of the total, with about 88% ($51.2 billion) of this discretionary funding going toward supporting VA health care programs, including medical and prosthetic research. The VA's mandatory budget authority accounted for about 51% ($63.8 billion) of the total VA budget authority, with about 80% ($51.2 billion) of this mandatory funding going toward disability compensation and pension programs. *Figure 2* provides a breakdown of the FY2013 President's budget request for both mandatory and discretionary programs (also see *Table 3*). For FY2013, the Administration is requesting approximately $135.6 billion. This includes approximately $61 billion in discretionary funding and nearly $74.6 billion in mandatory funding. According to the VA, the increase in mandatory funding over the FY2012-enacted amount could be attributed to increase in disability claims and the increase in readjustment benefits[22]

OVERVIEW OF VETERANS HEALTH ADMINISTRATION'S BUDGET FORMULATION[23]

Similar to most federal agencies, the VA begins formulating its budget request approximately 10 months before the President submits the budget to Congress in early February. VHA's budget request to Congress begins with the formulations of the budget based on the Enrollee Health Care Projection Model (EHCPM).[24] The model estimates the amount of budgetary resources VHA will need to meet the expected demand for most of the health care services it provides.

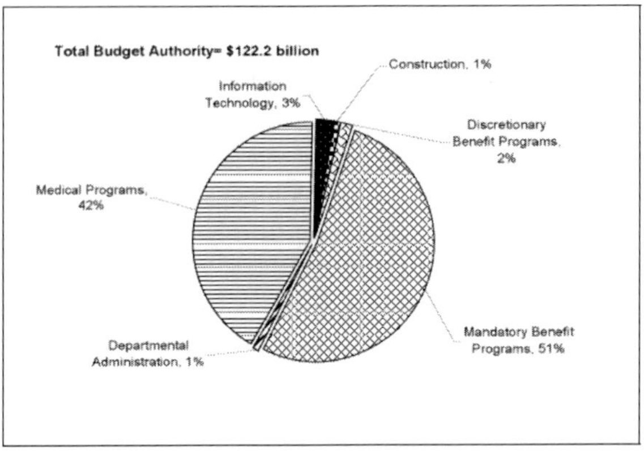

Source: Chart prepared by the Congressional Research Service based on H.Rept. 112-331.

Notes: Discretionary budget authority includes medical programs; information technology; construction; other discretionary benefits, such as operation and maintenance of VA's national cemeteries; and departmental administration. Mandatory benefits includes, disability compensation, pensions, education, vocational rehabilitation and employment services, among other benefits and services.

Figure 1. FY2012 VA Budget Allocations.

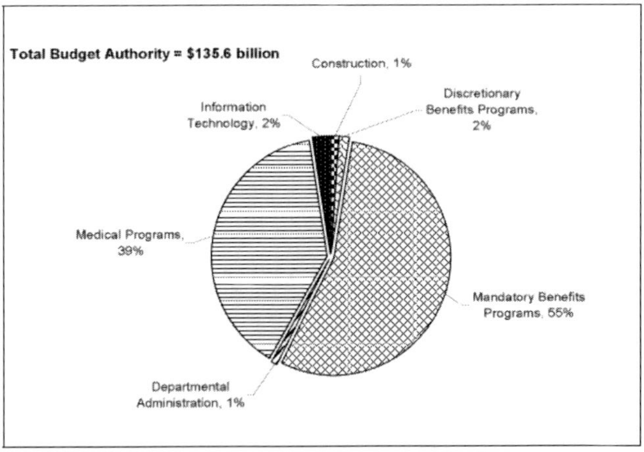

Source: Chart prepared by the Congressional Research Service based on Department of Veterans Affairs, FY2013 Budget Submission, Summary Volume, Volume 1 of 4, February 2012, p. 1B-1, and H.Rept. 112-491 and S.Rept. 112-168.

Figure 2. FY2013 VA Budget Request.

The EHCPM's estimates are based on three basic components: the projected number of veterans who will be enrolled in VA health care, the projected utilization of VA's health care services—that is, the quantity of health care services enrollees are expected to use—and the projected unit cost of providing these services. Each component is subject to a number of adjustments to account for the characteristics of VA health care and the veterans who access VA's health care services. The EHCPM makes projections three or four years into the future. Each year, VHA updates the EHCPM estimates to "incorporate the most recent data on health care utilization rates, actual program experience, and other factors, such as economic trends in unemployment and inflation."[25] For instance, in 2011, VHA used data from FY2010 to develop its health care budget estimate for the FY2013 request, including the advance appropriations request for FY2014.[26]

FUNDING FOR THE VHA

As noted previously, VHA is funded through four appropriations accounts. These are supplemented by other sources of revenue. Although the appropriations account structure has been subject to change from year to year, the appropriation accounts used to support the VHA traditionally include medical care, medical and prosthetic research, and medical administration. Congress also appropriates funds for construction of medical facilities through a larger appropriations account for construction for all VA facilities. In FY2004, "to provide better oversight and [to] receive a more accurate accounting of funds," Congress changed the VHA's appropriations structure.[27] Specifically, the Department of Veterans Affairs and Housing and Urban Development and Independent Agencies Appropriations Act, 2004 (P.L. 108-199, H.Rept. 108-401), funded VHA through four accounts: (1) medical services, (2) medical administration (currently known as medical support and compliance), (3) medical facilities, and (4) medical and prosthetic research. Brief descriptions of these accounts are provided below.

Medical Services

The medical services account covers expenses for furnishing inpatient and outpatient care and treatment of veterans and certain dependents, including care and treatment in non-VA facilities; outpatient care on a fee basis; medical supplies and equipment; salaries and expenses of employees hired under Title 38, United States Code (U.S.C.); cost of hospital food service operations;[28] aid to state veterans' homes; and assistance and support services for family caregivers of veterans authorized by the Caregivers and Veterans Omnibus Health Services Act of 2010 (P.L. 111-163). For FY2013, the President's budget request is proposing to transfer funding for biomedical engineering services from the medical facilities account to this account.[29]

Medical Support and Compliance (Previously Medical Administration)

This account provides for expenses related to the management, security, and administration of the VA health care system through the operation of VA medical centers, and other medical facilities such as community-based outpatient clinics (CBOCs)[30] and Vet Centers.[31] It also funds 21 Veterans Integrated Service Network (VISN)[32] offices and facility director offices; chief of staff operations; public health and environmental hazard programs; quality and performance management programs; medical inspection; human research oversight; training programs and continuing education; security; volunteer operations; and human resources management.

Medical Facilities

The medical facilities account funds expenses pertaining to the operations and maintenance of the VHA's capital infrastructure. These expenses include utilities and administrative expenses related to planning, designing, and executing construction or renovation projects at VHA facilities. It also funds leases, laundry services, grounds maintenance, trash removal, housekeeping, fire protection, pest management, and property disposition and acquisition.

Medical and Prosthetic Research

As required by law, the medical and prosthetic research program (medical research) focuses on research into the special health care needs of veterans.[33] This account provides funding for many types of research, such as investigator-initiated research; mentored research; large-scale, multi-site clinical trials; and centers of excellence. VA researchers receive funding not only through this account but also from the Department of Defense (DOD), the National Institutes of Health (NIH), and private sources.

In general, VA's research program is intramural; that is, research is performed by VA investigators at VA facilities and approved off-site locations. Unlike other federal agencies, such as NIH and DOD, VA does not have the statutory authority to make research grants to colleges and universities, cities and states, or any other non-VA entities.

Medical Care Collections Fund (MCCF)

In addition to direct appropriations accounts mentioned above, the Committees on Appropriations include medical care cost recovery collections when considering funding for the VHA. Congress has provided VHA the authority to bill some veterans and most health care insurers for nonservice-connected care provided to veterans enrolled in the VA health care system, to help defray the cost of delivering medical services to veterans.[34] Funds collected from first and third party (copayments and insurance) bills are retained by the VA health care facility that provided the care for the veteran.

Total MCCF revenue increased 25% over the past four fiscal years, from approximately $2.2 billion in FY2007 to nearly $2.8 billion in FY2011 (see *Table 1*). VHA is expecting MCCF total collections to approximate $2.8 billion in FY2012, although this amount is lower than MCCF collections in FY2009 and FY2010. Furthermore, total third-party revenue increased 42.7 % over the last four fiscal years from 1.3 billion in FY2007 to approximately 1.8 billion in FY2011. However, in FY2012 VHA expects lower first-party copayments. This estimated decline is "attributable to fewer veterans with billable insurance and increased numbers of veterans requesting hardship waivers and exemptions from first-party copayments."[35] Furthermore, VHA has stated that it continues to experience a decline in third-party collections "to billings ratios as commercial health insurers shift more responsibility to the patient for health care costs including copayments and deductibles, which VHA cannot collect."[36] It should noted that 38 U.S.C. §1729 prevents VHA from billing the veteran if the health insurer does not pay. Additionally, according to VHA, "FY2012 begins to reflect the shift in workload for Vietnam-era veterans aging to 65 years and older. Once a veteran is Medicare-eligible, Medicare becomes the primary insurance coverage and VA can bill insurance companies only for the portions Medicare does not cover (typically their deductibles). This significantly reduces the amount VA can collect."[37]

Table 1. Medical Care Collections, FY2007-FY2012 ($ in thousands)

	FY2007 Actual	FY2008 Actual	FY2009 Actual	FY2010 Actual	FY2011 Actual	FY2012 Estimate
First-party pharmacy copayments[a]	$760,616	$749,685	$720,238	$698,325	$729,742	$696,000
First-party copayments for inpatient andoutpatient care[b]	150,964	168,274	168,092	168,519	178,469	177,000
First-party long-term care copayments[c]	3,699	3,751	3,419	3,092	3,174	4,000
Subtotal first-party copayments	915,279	921,710	891,749	869,936	911,385	877,000
Third-party insurance collections[d]	1,261,346	1,497,449	1,843,202	1,904,032	1,799,951	1,825,000
Enhanced use leasing revenue[e]	1,692	1,422	1,601	1,694	1,398	2,000
Compensated work therapy collections[f]	43,296	52,372	56,106	57,108	55,099	57,000
Parking fees[g]	3,136	3,355	3,585	3,611	3,842	4,000
Compensation and pension living expenses[h]	1,904	1,572	1,952	1,523	871	2,000
MCCF Total	$2,226,653	$2,477,880	$2,798,195	2,837,904	2,772,546	2,767,000

Source: Table prepared by the Congressional Research Service based on figures obtained from the Department of Veterans Affairs, FY2009-2013 Congressional Budget Submissions.

a. In FY2002, Congress created the Health Services Improvement Fund (HSIF) to collect increases in pharmacy copayments (from $2 to $7 for a 30-day supply of outpatient medication; currently $8 for Priority Groups 2-6 veterans and $9 for Priority Groups 7 and 8 veterans), which went into effect on February 4, 2002. The Consolidated Appropriations Resolution, 2003 (P.L. 108-7) granted the VA the authority to consolidate the HSIF with the MCCF and granted permanent authority to recover copayments for outpatient medications.

b. Authorized at 38 U.S.C. §1710(f) and 1710(g).

c. Authority to collect long-term care copayments was established by the Millennium Health Care and Benefits Act (P.L. 106-117). Certain veteran patients receiving extended care services from VA providers or outside contractors are charged copayments. The Caregivers and Veterans Omnibus Health Services Act of 2010 (P.L. 111-163) extended the authority to collect copayments for nursing home care through September 30, 2012.

d. Authorized at 38 U.S.C. §1729(a).

e. Under the enhanced-use lease authority, the VA may lease land or buildings to the private sector for up to 75 years. In return the VA receives fair consideration in cash and/or in-kind. Funds received as monetary considerations may be used to provide care for veterans.

f. The compensated work therapy program is a comprehensive rehabilitation program that prepares veterans for competitive employment and independent living. As part of their work therapy, veterans produce items for sale or undertake subcontracts to provide certain products and/or services, such as providing temporary staffing to a private firm. Funds collected from the sale of these products and/or services are deposited into the MCCF.

g. The Parking program provides funds for construction and acquisition of parking garages at VA medical facilities. The VA collects fees for use of these parking facilities.

h. Under the compensation and pension living expenses program, veterans who do not have either a spouse or child would have their monthly pension reduced to $90 after the third month a veteran is admitted for nursing home care. The difference between the veteran's pension and the $90 is used for the operation of the VA medical facility.

FY2012 Budget Summary[38]

President's Request

The President submitted his FY2012 budget request to Congress on February 14, 2011. The Administration's FY2012 budget request for VHA (medical services, medical support and compliance, medical facilities, and medical and prosthetic research) was $51.4 billion. The President's budget proposed to set up a $953 million contingency fund that would have provided additional funds up to $953 million to become available for obligation if the Administration determined that additional funds were required due to changes in economic conditions in 2012. Furthermore, as required by the Veterans Health Care Budget Reform and Transparency Act of 2009 (P.L. 111-81), the President's budget requested $52.5 billion in advance appropriations for the three medical care accounts (medical services, medical support and compliance, and medical facilities) for FY2013 (*Table 2*).

House and Senate Action

On June 14, the House passed the Military Construction and Veterans Affairs and Related Agencies Appropriations bill (MILCON-VA Appropriations bill) for FY2012 (H.R. 2055; H.Rept. 112-94). The House-passed measure provided $51.1 billion for VHA for FY2012 (*Table 2*). The Senate passed its version of the MILCON-VA Appropriations bill for FY2012 (H.R. 2055; S.Rept. 112-29) on July 20. The Senate-passed version of H.R. 2055 provided a total of $51.2 billion for VHA (*Table 2).* The House- and Senate-passed versions of the MILCON-VA Appropriations bill for FY2012 provided $52.5 billion in advance appropriations for FY2013. Furthermore, both the House and Senate versions of the MILCON-VA Appropriations bill for FY2012 (H.Rept. 112-94; S.Rept. 112-29) did not approve the President's proposal to set up a $953 million contingency fund.

Consolidated Appropriations Act, 2012

Congress did not pass the MILCON-VA Appropriations bill for FY2012 before the fiscal year began on October 1, 2011, and funded most of the VA through a series of short-term continuing resolutions (CRs). On December 15, 2011, House and Senate conferees of H.R. 2055 reported a conference agreement (H.Rept. 112-331), which was titled the Consolidated Appropriations Act, 2012, and included nine appropriations bills. Division H of this measure contained the MILCONVA Appropriations Act, 2012. The Consolidated Appropriations Act, 2012 (P.L. 112-74; H.Rept. 112-331), was enacted into law on December 23, 2011. P.L. 112-74 provides a total of $51.2 billion for VHA for FY2012 and $52.5 billion in advance appropriations for FY2013 (*Table 2*). The Consolidated Appropriations Act, 2012 (P.L. 112-74), did not include the President's proposal to set up a $953 million contingency fund.

Table 2. VHA Appropriations, by Account, FY2011-FY2012, and Advance Appropriations, FY2013 ($ in thousands)

	Full-Year Continuing Appropriations Act, 2011 (H.R. 1473; P.L. 112-10)		President's Budget Request		House (H.R. 2055; H.Rept. 112-94)		Senate (H.R. 2055; S.Rept. 112-29)		Consolidated Appropriations Act, 2012 (P.L. 112-74; H.Rept. 112-331)	
Account	FY2011[a]	FY2012	FY2012	FY2013	FY2012	FY2013	FY2012	FY2013	FY2012	FY2013
Medical Services	$37,061,728	—	$39,649,985	—	$39,649,985	—	$39,649,985	—	$39,649,985	—
Additional Funding over FY2012 Advance Appropriation	—	—	$240,000	—	—	—	—	—	—	—
Subtotal Medical Services	37,061,728	—	39,889,985	—	39,649,985	—	39,649,985	—	39,649,985	—
Medical Support and Compliance (Previously Medical Administration)	5,296,454	—	5,535,000	—	5,535,000	—	5,535,000	—	5,535,000	—
Pay Freeze Rescission (P.L. 112-10)	-34,000	—	—	—	—	—	—	—	—	—

Table 2. (Continued)

	Full-Year Continuing Appropriations Act, 2011 (H.R. 1473; P.L. 112-10)		President's Budget Request		House (H.R. 2055; H.Rept. 112-94)		Senate (H.R. 2055; S.Rept. 112-29)		Consolidated Appropriations Act, 2012 (P.L. 112-74; H.Rept. 112-331)	
Account	FY2011[a]	FY2012	FY2012	FY2013	FY2012	FY2013	FY2012	FY2013	FY2012	FY2013
Subtotal Medical Support and Compliance (Previously Medical Administration)	5,262,454	—	5,535,000	—	5,535,000	—	5,535,000	—	5,535,000	—
Medical Facilities	5,728,550	—	5,426,000	—	5,426,000	—	5,426,000	—	5,426,000	—
Pay Freeze Rescission (P.L. 112-10)	-15,000	—	—	—	—	—	—	—	—	—
Subtotal Medical Facilities	5,713,550	—	5,426,000	—	5,426,000	—	5,426,000	—	5,426,000	—
Medical and Prosthetic Research	579,838	—	508,774	—	530,774	—	581,000	—	581,000	—
Subtotal Medical and Prosthetic Research	579,838	—	508,774	—	530,774	—	581,000	—	581,000	—

	Full-Year Continuing Appropriations Act, 2011 (H.R. 1473; P.L. 112-10)		President's Budget Request		House (H.R. 2055; H.Rept. 112-94)		Senate (H.R. 2055; S.Rept. 112-29)		Consolidated Appropriations Act, 2012 (P.L. 112-74; H.Rept. 112-331)	
Account	FY2011[a]	FY2012	FY2012	FY2013	FY2012	FY2013	FY2012	FY2013	FY2012	FY2013
Total VHA Appropriations (without collections)	48,617,570	—	51,359,759	—	51,141,759	—	51,191,985	—	51,191,985	—
Medical Care Cost Collections (MCCF)	3,393,000	—	$3,326,000	—	3,326,000	—	3,326,000	—	3,326,000	—
Total VHA Appropriations (with collections)	$52,010,570	—	$54,685,759	—	$54,467,759	—	$54,517,985	—	$54,517,985	—
Memorandum: Advance Appropriations[b]										
Medical Services	—	$39,649,985	—	$41,354,000	—	$41,354,000	—	$41,354,000	—	$41,354,000
Medical Support and Compliance (Previously Medical Administration)	—	5,535,000	—	$5,746,000	—	5,746,000	—	5,746,000	—	5,746,000
Medical Facilities	—	5,426,000	—	$5,441,000	—	5,441,000	—	5,441,000	—	5,441,000

Table 2. (Continued)

	Full-Year Continuing Appropriations Act, 2011 (H.R. 1473; P.L. 112-10)		President's Budget Request		House (H.R. 2055; H.Rept. 112-94)		Senate (H.R. 2055; S.Rept. 112-29)		Consolidated Appropriations Act, 2012 (P.L. 112-74; H.Rept. 112-331)	
Account	FY2011[a]	FY2012	FY2012	FY2013	FY2012	FY2013	FY2012	FY2013	FY2012	FY2013
Total VHA Appropriations	—	$50,610,985	—	$52,541,000	—	$52,541,000	—	$52,541,000	—	$52,541,000

Source: Prepared by the Congressional Research Service. FY2011 enacted figures based on information from the House Committee on Appropriations, Subcommittee on Military Construction, Veterans Affairs, and Related Agencies, and S.Rept. 112-29. FY2012 request and House and Senate figures based on H.Rept. 112-94, and S.Rept. 112- 29. Final enacted numbers for FY2012 based on H.Rept. 112-331.

[a] This amount also reflects the 0.2% government-wide rescission required by Division B, Section 1119(a) of the Department of Defense and Full-Year Continuing Appropriations Act, 2011 (P.L. 112-10), and the FY2011 pay freeze rescission.

[b] The Veterans Health Care Budget Reform and Transparency Act 2009 (P.L. 111-81; codified at 38 U.S.C. §117) provided for advance appropriations (appropriations that become available one fiscal year after the fiscal year for which the appropriations act was enacted) for VA's medical services, medical support and compliance, and medical facilities appropriations accounts, and requires the VA to submit a request for advance appropriation with its budget submission year. The Department of Defense and Full-Year Continuing Appropriations Act, 2011 (P.L. 112-10) provided budget authority for FY2012 for the following accounts: medical services, medical support and compliance, and medical facilities. Under current budget scoring guidelines new budget authority for an advance appropriation is scored in the fiscal year in which the funds become available for obligation. Therefore, in this table the budget authority is recorded in the FY2012 column. Likewise, the Consolidated Appropriations Act, 2012 (P.L. 112-74 (H.Rept. 112-331) provided advance appropriations budget authority for FY2013 for those same accounts. Under current budget scoring guidelines, new budget authority for an advance appropriation is scored in the fiscal year in which the funds become available for obligation. Therefore, in this table this budget authority is recorded in the FY2013 column.

FY2013 VHA BUDGET

President's Request

The Obama Administration's FY2013 budget request was submitted to Congress on February 13, 2012. The President's budget is requesting $135.6 billion in budget authority for the VA as a whole. This includes approximately $75 billion in mandatory funding and $61 billion in discretionary funding (*Table 3*). For FY2013, the Administration requests $53.3 billion (excluding estimated MCCF collections) for VHA. This includes $41.5 billion for the medical services account, $5.7 billion for the medical support and compliance account, $5.4 billion for the medical facilities account, and nearly $583 million for the medical and prosthetic research account (*Table 4*). The total request for VHA represents a 4.1% increase over the FY2012- enacted appropriations. According to the VA, this increase reflects the increased costs of the implementation of the Caregivers and Veterans Omnibus Health Services Act (P.L. 111-163), and the Agent Orange[39] and Amyotrophic Lateral Sclerosis (ALS) presumptions established by the VA.[40]

As required by the Veterans Health Care Budget Reform and Transparency Act of 2009 (P.L. 111- 81), the President's budget is requesting $54.5 billion in advance appropriations for the three medical care appropriations (medical services, medical support and compliance, and medical facilities) for FY2014, an increase of approximately 3.7% over the FY2013-enacted amount of $52.5 billion for the same three accounts. In FY2014, the Administration's budget request would provide $43.6 billion for the medical services account, $6.0 billion for the medical support and compliance account, and $4.9 billion for the medical facilities account (*Table 4*).

Budget Control Act of 2011 (BCA, P.L. 112-25) and VHA Appropriations

It should be noted that the House and Senate appropriators will be considering FY2013 discretionary appropriations in the context of the Budget Control Act of 2011.

The Budget Control Act of 2011 (BCA, P.L. 112-25) contained an overall discretionary spending cap for FY2013 of $1.047 trillion. On March 29, 2012, the House passed a budget resolution (H.Con.Res. 112) that caps spending at a lower level, $1.028 trillion. The Senate has not passed a budget resolution, but on April 19 the Senate Appropriations Committee allotted subcommittee funding levels that were equal to the total $1.047 trillion cap in the BCA.

Budget Control Act of 2011 (BCA, P.L. 112-25) and VHA Appropriations

FY2013 discretionary appropriations will be considered in the context of the Budget Control Act of 2011 (BCA, P.L. 112-25), which established discretionary spending limits for FY2012-FY2021. The BCA also tasked a Joint Select Committee on Deficit Reduction to develop a federal deficit reduction plan for Congress and the President to enact by January 15, 2012. The failure of Congress and the President to enact deficit reduction legislation by that date triggered an automatic spending reduction process established by the BCA, consisting of a combination of sequestration and lower discretionary spending caps, to begin on January 2, 2013. The sequestration process for FY2013 requires across-the-board spending cuts at the account and program level to achieve equal budget reductions from both defense and nondefense funding at a percentage to be determined, under terms specified in the Balanced Budget and Emergency Deficit Control Act of 1985 (BBEDCA, Title II of P.L. 99-177, 2 U.S.C. 900-922), as amended by the BCA, by the Office of Management and Budget.

Certain programs are exempt from sequestration, and special rules govern the sequestration of others. For the most part, these provisions are found in Sections 255 and 256 of the Balanced Budget and Emergency Deficit Control Act (BBEDCA Title II of P.L. 99-177, 2 U.S.C. 900-922), as amended. Section 255 of BBEDCA, as amended in 2010 (P.L. 111-139), specifically excludes from sequestration, among other programs, appropriations for all programs administered by the VA. Nevertheless, Section 256(e) of BBEDCA appears to allow a maximum 2% reduction in budget authority for VA medical care for any fiscal year. This apparent discrepancy between the two sections of the law raised questions about whether VA will be totally exempt from sequestration or whether medical care will be subject to a maximum permissible 2% reduction in budget authority, if sequestration occurs as scheduled on January 2, 2013. On April 23, 2012, OMB issued a letter stating that "all programs administered by the VA, including Veterans' Medicare Care, are exempt from sequestration under Section 255(b)."[41]

House Budget Resolution

On March 20, 2012, the Chairman of the House Budget Committee released the Chairman's mark of the FY2013 House budget resolution. The House Budget Committee considered the Chairman's mark on March 21, 2012, and voted to report the budget resolution to the full House. H.Con.Res. 112 was introduced in the House March 23, 2012, and was accompanied by the House Budget Committee report (H.Rept. 112-421). The House passed H.Con.Res. 112 on March 29, 2012. According to the Committee report to accompany H.Con.Res 112:

> The resolution calls for $134.6 billion in budget authority and $135.2 billion in outlays in fiscal year 2013.... Discretionary spending is $61.3 billion in budget authority and $62.1 billion in outlays in fiscal year 2013. This resolution also provides for up to $54.5 billion in advance appropriations for medical care, consistent with the Veterans Health Care Budget and Reform Transparency Act of 2009. Mandatory spending in 2013 is $73.3 billion in budget authority and $73.2 billion in outlays.[42]

House Action

On May 8, 2012, the House Military Construction and Veterans Affairs Subcommittee approved its version of a Military Construction and Veterans Affairs and Related Agencies Appropriations bill for FY2013 (MILCON-VA Appropriations bill). The full House Appropriations Committee voted to report the measure on May 16, and the House passed H.R. 5854 on May 31. The MILCON-VA Appropriations bill for FY2013 (H.R. 5854; H.Rept. 112-491) provides a total of $135.4 billion for the VA. This amount is $13.2 billion (10.8%) above the FY2012-enacted amount of 122.2 billion and 0.2% below the President's request of $135.6 billion for FY2013 (*Table 3*).

H.R. 5854 (H.Rept. 112-491) as passed by the House provides $53.1 billion for VHA, which comprises four accounts: medical services, medical support and compliance, medical facilities, and medical and prosthetic research. The total amount for VHA is approximately $2.0 billion above the FY2012-enacted amount and 0.3% less than the Administration's budget request for FY2013 (*Table 4*).

During committee mark up of the MILCON-VA Appropriations bill, the House Appropriations Committee noted with concern VHA's revision of budget estimates for FY2012 and FY2013 and the lack of timely notification to the Appropriation Committees. According to the President's budget submission in February 2012, there had been a significant revision to both the FY2012 and FY2013 VHA budget estimates. This revision occurred after VHA ran its Enrollee Healthcare Projection Model in the spring of 2011 using updated information. The result of this update was a lowering of appropriations for VHA in FY2012 by nearly $3 billion, and nearly $2 billion for FY2013. VHA subsequently made an internal decision to reallocate those resources to fund a variety of initiatives.

To address this lapse of notification to Congress, the committee included bill language requiring the VHA to notify the Congress of any changes in funding requirements exceeding $250 million identified when the Enrollee Healthcare Projection Model is recalculated in the spring of each year. Additionally, H.R. 5854 contains bill language requiring the VHA to submit a reprogramming request when it proposes a change in funding for initiatives listed on the "VA Medical Care Obligations by Program" page in the President's budget submission to Congress.[43]

Medical Services

The MILCON-VA Appropriations bill provides $41.4 billion for the medical services account for FY2013. The FY2013 budget request included a request for an additional $165 million for this account for FY2013. The House-passed measure did not provide this additional amount of funding. According to the committee report to accompany H.R. 5854, "[S]ince the VA has significantly overestimated Medical Care funding needs for both [FY] 2012 and [FY] 2013, the Committee is reluctant to provide any additional 2013 funding at this time. Should any shortfall occur, the Department should utilize funding from administrative expenses for VHA headquarters and the veterans integrated service networks (VISNs)."[44]

As required by the Veterans Health Care Budget Reform and Transparency Act of 2009 (P.L. 111- 81), H.R. 5854 provides $43.6 billion in advance appropriations for the medical services account for FY2014, an increase of 2.2 billion over the FY2013 amount, and the same as the budget request (*Table 4*).

During floor debate on the MILCON-VA Appropriations bill for FY2013, several amendments were offered that sought to designate in debate funds for certain purposes. H.Amdt. 1159, as agreed by the House, designates $16 million within the Office of Rural Health to expand the pilot program known as Access Received Closer to Home (Project ARCH).[45]

Medical Support and Compliance

The MILCON-VA Appropriations bill (H.R. 5854) provides $5.7 billion for this account for FY2013, same as the Administration's request and $211 million above the FY2012-enacted amount (*Table 4*). The bill also provides $6.0 billion in advance appropriations for FY2014 for this account, same as the requested amount.

Medical Facilities

H.R. 5854 provides $5.4 billion for this account for FY2013, which is $15 million above the FY2012-enacted amount. The House Appropriations Committee reported bill recommends an advance appropriation of approximately $4.9 billion for FY2014, a decrease of $569 million below the FY2013 level, and same the President's request.

Medical and Prosthetic Research

The MILCON-VA Appropriations bill (H.R. 5854) appropriates approximately $582.7 million for this account, an increase of $1.7 million above the FY2012-enacted amount and same as the Administration's request.

During floor consideration of H.R. 5854 another amendment, H.Amdt. 1158, was agreed to by the House. H.Amdt. 1158 designates $35 million of the medical and prosthetic research account for Post-traumatic Stress Disorder (PTSD) and Traumatic Brain Injury (TBI) research.[46]

Senate Committee Action

The Senate Appropriations Committee, Military Construction, Veterans Affairs Subcommittee approved its version of a draft MILCON-VA Appropriations bill on May 15, 2012; the full Senate Appropriations Committee reported the draft measure on May 22. The Senate Appropriations Committee-reported MILCON-VA Appropriations bill (S. 3215; S.Rept. 112-168) provides a total of $135.6 billion for VA, same as the President's request, and $13.4 billion above the FY2012- enacted amount (*Table 3*).

The MILCON-VA Appropriations bill (S. 3215; S.Rept. 112-168) provides $53.3 billion for VHA for FY2013, which comprises four accounts: medical services, medical support and compliance, medical facilities, and medical and prosthetic research. The total amount for VHA is approximately $2.1 billion above the FY2012-enacted amount and $10 million less than the Administration's request (*Table 4*).

Medical Services

The MILCON-VA Appropriations bill (S. 3215; S.Rept. 112-168) appropriates $41.5 billion for this account, this amount is $10 million less than the Administration's request for FY2013. S. 3215 also includes an advance appropriation of $43.6 billion for medical services for FY2014. This is $2.0 above FY2013 and equal to the FY2014 budget request. According to the committee report, FY2013 appropriation includes $6.2 billion for mental healthcare; $72.8 million for suicide prevention; $3.2 million to provide medical care to Afghanistan and Iraq war veterans; $222 million for readjustment counseling services at Vet Centers; $2.6 billion for prosthetics; and $1.4 billion for specific homeless veterans programs.[47]

Medical Support and Compliance

S. 3215 provides $5.7 billion for FY2013 for this account. This is $211 million above the FY2012-enacted level and equal to the budget request. Additionally, the bill includes an advance appropriation of $6.0 billion for FY2014, which is $287 million above FY2013 and equal to the Administration's request.

Medical Facilities

The MILCON-VA Appropriations bill (S. 3215; S.Rept. 112-168) appropriates $5.4 billion for FY2013 for the medical facilities account. The bill also includes an advance appropriation of $4.9 billon for FY2014. This is $569 million below the FY2013 level and equal to the President's request. According to S.Rept. 112-168, in FY2014, the VHA will transfer 1,080 full-time personnel currently budgeted for in this account to the medical services account. The committee report states that "while this transfer accounts for a reduction of $320,000,000 in the Medical facilities account and a respective increase in the Medical services account, it does not fully explain the decline in the Medical facilities account."[48]

Medical and Prosthetic Research

The MILCON-VA Appropriations bill (S. 3215) appropriates approximately $582.7 million for this account, an increase of $1.7 million above the FY2012-enacted amount and same as the Administration's request.

Table 3. VA Appropriations, FY2012-FY2013, and Advance Appropriations, FY2014 ($ in thousands)

	Consolidated Appropriations Act, 2012 (P.L. 112-74; H.Rept. 112-331)		President's Budget Request		House (H.R. 5854; H.Rept. 112-491)		Senate Committee (S. 3215; S.Rept. 112-168)	
	FY2012	FY2013	FY2013	FY2014	FY2013	FY2014	FY2013	FY2014
Total Department of Veterans Affairs (VA)	$122,226,272	—	$135,636,648	—	$135,377,850[a]	—	$135,636,648	—
Total Mandatory	63,764,919	—	74,638,167	—	74,638,167	—	74,638,167	—
Total Discretionary	58,461,353	—	60,998,481	—	60,739,683	—	60,998,481	—
Total Veterans Health Administration (VHA)[b]	$51,191,985	—	$53,288,674	—	$53,123,674	—	$53,278,674	—
Memorandum: Advance appropriations VHA[c]	—	$52,541,000	—	$54,462,000	—	$54,462,000	—	$54,462,000

Source: Table prepared by the Congressional Research Service. The FY2012 final enacted numbers are based on H.Rept. 112-331. FY2013 House and Senate figures and FY2014 advance appropriations figures are based on H.Rept. 112-491; S.Rept. 112-168; and Congressional Record, daily edition, vol. 158 (May 31, 2012), pp. H3311-H3314.

[a] This amount reflects the 0.5% rescission of the Federal employee pay raise (The House-passed measure did not provide funding for the 0.5% percent Federal employee pay raise assumed in the President's budget request).

[b] Includes funding for medical services, medical support and compliance, medical facilities, and medical and prosthetic research accounts, and excludes collections deposited into the Medical Care Collections Fund (MCCF).

[c] The Veterans Health Care Budget Reform and Transparency Act 2009 (P.L. 111-81; codified at 38 U.S.C. §117) provided for advance appropriations (appropriations that become available one fiscal year after the fiscal year for which the appropriations act was enacted) for VA's medical services, medical support and compliance, and medical facilities appropriations accounts, and requires the VA to submit a request for advance appropriation with its budget submission year. The Consolidated Appropriations Act, 2012 (P.L. 112-74; H.Rept. 112-331) provided advance appropriations budget authority for FY2013 for the following accounts: medical services, medical support and compliance, and medical facilities. Under current budget scoring guidelines new budget authority for an advance appropriation is scored in the fiscal year in which the funds become available for obligation. Therefore, in this table the budget authority is recorded in the FY2013 column. The Administration's advance appropriations request for FY2014 and the House-passed and the Senate Appropriations Committee recommended amounts are recorded in the FY2014 column.

Table 4. VHA Appropriations by Account, FY2012-FY2013, and Advance Appropriations, FY2014 ($ in thousands)

	Consolidated Appropriations Act, 2012 (P.L. 112-74; H.Rept. 112-331)		President's Budget Request		House (H.R. 5854; H.Rept. 112-491)		Senate Committee (S. 3215; S.Rept. 112-168)	
Account	FY2012	FY2013	FY2013	FY2014	FY2013	FY2014	FY2013	FY2014
Medical Services	$39,649,985	—	$41,354,000	—	$41,354,000	—	$41,354,000	—
Additional Funding over FY2013 Advance Appropriation	—	—	165,000	—	—	—	155,000	
Subtotal Medical Services	39,649,985	—	41,519,000	—	41,354,000	—	41,509,000	—
Medical Support and Compliance (Previously Medical Administration)	5,535,000	—	5,746,000	—	5,746,000	—	5,746,000	—
Subtotal Medical Support and Compliance (Previously Medical Administration)	5,535,000	—	5,746,000	—	5,746,000	—	5,746,000	—
Medical Facilities	5,426,000	—	5,441,000	—	5,441,000	—	5,441,000	—
Subtotal Medical Facilities	5,426,000	—	5,441,000	—	5,441,000	—	5,441,000	—

	Consolidated Appropriations Act, 2012 (P.L. 112-74; H.Rept. 112-331)		President's Budget Request		House (H.R. 5854; H.Rept. 112-491)		Senate Committee (S. 3215; S.Rept. 112-168)	
Account	FY2012	FY2013	FY2013	FY2014	FY2013	FY2014	FY2013	FY2014
Medical and Prosthetic Research	581,000	—	582,674	—	582,674	—	582,674	—
Subtotal Medical and Prosthetic Research	581,000	—	582,674	—	582,674	—	582,674	—
Total VHA Appropriations (without collections)	51,191,985	—	53,288,674	—	53,123,674[a]	—	53,278,674	—
Medical Care Cost Collections (MCCF)	3,326,000	—	2,527,000	—	2,527,000	—	2,527,000	—
Total VHA Appropriations (with collections)	$54,517,985	—	$55,815,674	—	$55,650,674	—	$55,805,674	—
Memorandum:								
Advance								
Appropriations[b]								
Medical Services	—	$41,354,000	—	$43,557,000	—	$43,557,000	—	$43,557,000
Medical Support and Compliance (Previously Medical Administration)	—	5,746,000	—	6,033,000	—	6,033,000	—	6,033,000

Table 4. (Continued)

	Consolidated Appropriations Act, 2012 (P.L. 112-74; H.Rept. 112-331)		President's Budget Request		House (H.R. 5854; H.Rept. 112-491)		Senate Committee (S. 3215; S.Rept. 112-168)	
Account	FY2012	FY2013	FY2013	FY2014	FY2013	FY2014	FY2013	FY2014
Medical Facilities	—	5,441,000	—	4,872,000	—	4,872,000	—	4,872,000
Total VHA Appropriations	—	$52,541,000	—	$54,462,000	—	$54,462,000	—	$54,462,000

Source: Table prepared by the Congressional Research Service. Final enacted numbers for FY2012 based on H.Rept. 112-331. FY2013 House and Senate figures and FY2014 advance appropriations figures are based on H.Rept. 112-491; S.Rept. 112-168; and Congressional Record, daily edition, vol. 158 (May 31, 2012), pp. H3311-H3314.

[a] This amount does not reflect the 0.5% rescission of the Federal employee pay raise (The House-passed measure did not provide funding for the 0.5% percent Federal employee pay raise assumed in the President's budget request).

[b] The Veterans Health Care Budget Reform and Transparency Act 2009 (P.L. 111-81; codified at 38 U.S.C. §117) provided for advance appropriations (appropriations that become available one fiscal year after the fiscal year for which the appropriations act was enacted) for VA's medical services, medical support and compliance, and medical facilities appropriations accounts, and requires the VA to submit a request for advance appropriation with its budget submission year. The Consolidated Appropriations Act, 2012 (P.L. 112-74; H.Rept. 112-331) provided advance appropriations budget authority for FY2013 for the following accounts: medical services, medical support and compliance, and medical facilities. Under current budget scoring guidelines new budget authority for an advance appropriation is scored in the fiscal year in which the funds become available for obligation. Therefore, in this table the budget authority is recorded in the FY2013 column. The Administration's advance appropriations request for FY2014 and the House-passed (H.R. 5854) and Senate Appropriations Committee recommended amounts(S.Rept. 112-168) are recorded in the FY2014 column.

State Veterans' Nursing Homes

The MILCON-VA Appropriations bill (S. 3215; S.Rept. 112-168) also includes an administrative provision that would provide VHA more flexibility in determining reimbursement rates for state veterans' nursing homes. Under this provision VHA would enter into contracts or agreements with state veterans' nursing homes for the care of any veteran with a service-connected disability rated 70% or more. The Veterans Benefits, Health Care, and Information Technology Act of 2006 (P.L. 109-461) required VHA to reimburse state veterans' nursing homes the cost of care of 70% or more service-connected disabled veterans. However, according to the National Association of State Veterans' Homes, the rates established by VHA under P.L. 109-461 did not reimburse state veterans' nursing homes adequately for the skilled nursing care of service-connected disabled veterans. Therefore, some state veterans' nursing homes either incurred losses or limited the admission veterans to minimize their financial losses.[49] Therefore, this administrative provision in the MILCON-VA Appropriations bill (S. 3215) is designed to remedy this situation.

APPENDIX A. VA PRIORITY GROUPS AND THEIR ELIGIBILITY CRITERIA

Table A-1. VA Priority Groups and Their Eligibility Criteria

Priority Group 1

Veterans with service-connected disabilities rated 50% or more disabling

Veterans determined by VA to be unemployable due to service-connected conditions

Priority Group 2

Veterans with service-connected disabilities rated 30% or 40% disabling

Priority Group 3

Veterans who are former POWs[a]

Veterans awarded the Purple Heart[b]

Veterans in receipt of the Medal of Honor[c]

Veterans whose discharge was for a disability that was incurred or aggravated in the line of duty

Veterans with service-connected disabilities rated 10% or 20% disabling

Veterans awarded special eligibility classification under Title 38, U.S.C., Section 1151, "benefits for individuals disabled by treatment or vocational rehabilitation"

Priority Group 4

Veterans who are receiving aid and attendance or housebound benefits Veterans who have been determined by VA to be catastrophically disabled

Priority Group 5

Nonservice-connected veterans and noncompensable service-connected veterans rated 0% disabled whose annual income and net worth are below the established VA means test thresholds

Veterans receiving VA pension benefits

Veterans eligible for Medicaid benefits

Priority Group 6

Compensable 0% service-connected veterans

Mexican Border War veterans

Veterans solely seeking care for disorders associated with

—exposure to herbicides while serving in Vietnam; or

—ionizing radiation during atmospheric testing or during the occupation of Hiroshima and Nagasaki; or

—for disorders associated with service in the Gulf War; or

—for any illness associated with service in combat in a war after the Gulf War or during a period of hostility after November 11, 1998 as follows:

- Veterans discharged from active duty on or after January 28, 2003, who were enrolled as of January 28, 2008, and veterans who apply for enrollment after January 28, 2008, for five years post discharge

-Veterans discharged from active duty before January 28, 2003, who apply for enrollment after January 28, 2008, until January 27, 2011

Priority Group 7

Veterans who agree to pay specified copayments with income and/or net worth above the VA means test threshold and income below the VA national geographic income thresholds

Priority Group 8

Veterans who agree to pay specified copayments with income and/or net worth above the VA means test threshold and the VA national geographic threshold

Subpriority a: Noncompensable 0% service-connected and enrolled as of January 16, 2003, and who have remained enrolled since that date and/or placed in this subpriority due to changed eligibility status

Subpriority b: Noncompensable 0% service-connected and enrolled on or after June 15, 2009, whose income exceeds the current VA means test threshold or VA national geographic income thresholds by 10% or less

Subpriority c: Nonservice-connected veterans enrolled as of January 16, 2003, and who have remained enrolled since that date and/or placed in this subpriority due to changed eligibility status

Subpriority d: Nonservice-connected veterans enrolled on or after June 15, 2009, whose income exceeds the current VA means test threshold or VA national geographic income thresholds by 10% or less

Subpriority e: Noncompensable 0% service-connected veterans not meeting the above criteria Subpriority g: Nonservice-connected veterans not meeting the above criteria

Source: Department of Veterans Affairs.

Notes: Service-connected disability means with respect to disability, that such disability was incurred or aggravated in the line of duty in the active military, naval or air service

[a] Veterans who are former Prisoners of War (POWs) are placed in Priority Group 3. This change occurred with the enactment of the Former Prisoner of War Benefits Act of 1981(P.L. 97-37) on August 14, 1981.

[b] Veterans in receipt of a Purple Heart are in Priority Group 3. This change occurred with the enactment of the Veterans Millennium Health Care and Benefits Act (P.L. 106-117) on November 30, 1999.

[c] Veterans in receipt of the Medal of Honor are in Priority Group 3. This change occurred with the enactment of the Caregiver and Veterans Omnibus Health Services Act of 2010 (P.L. 111-163) on May 5, 2010.

End Notes

[1] In general, payments of benefits made to, or on account of, a beneficiary under any law administered by the VA are exempt from federal taxation (38 U.S.C. §5301).

[2] For a detailed description of disability compensation and pension programs see, CRS Report R42324, "Who is a Veteran?"—Basic Eligibility for Veterans' Benefits, by Christine Scott; CRS Report RL34626, Veterans' Benefits: Benefits Available for Disabled Veterans, by Christine Scott, Carol D. Davis, and Libby Perl; and CRS Report RS22804, Veterans' Benefits: Pension Benefit Programs, by Christine Scott and Carol D. Davis.

[3] For a discussion of education benefits, see CRS Report R40723, Educational Assistance Programs Administered by the U.S. Department of Veterans Affairs, by Cassandria Dortch.

[4] For details on VA's vocational rehabilitation and employment see, CRS Report RL34627, Veterans' Benefits: The Vocational Rehabilitation and Employment Program, by Benjamin Collins.

[5] For detailed information on homeless veterans programs see, CRS Report RL34024, Veterans and Homelessness, by Libby Perl.

[6] For details on guaranteed loans, direct loans, and specially adapted housing grants see, CRS Report R42504, VA Housing: Guaranteed Loans, Direct Loans, and Specially Adapted Housing Grants, by Libby Perl.

[7] For details on insurance programs see, CRS Report R41435, Veterans' Benefits: Current Life Insurance Programs, by Christine Scott.

[8] For details on death benefits, see CRS Report R41386, Veterans' Benefits: Burial Benefits and National Cemeteries, by Christine Scott.

[9] Established by the National Cemeteries Act of 1973 (P.L. 93-43).

[10] Veteran's status is established by active-duty status in the U.S. Armed Forces and an honorable discharge or release from active military service. Generally, persons enlisting in one of the armed forces after September 7, 1980, and officers commissioned after October 16, 1981, must have completed two years of active duty or the full period of their initial service obligation to be eligible for VA health care benefits. Servicemembers discharged at any time because of service-connected disabilities are not held to this requirement.

[11] A service-connected disability is a disability that was incurred or aggravated in the line of duty in the U.S. Armed Forces (38 U.S.C. §101 (16), VA determines whether veterans have service-connected disabilities, and for those with such disabilities, assigns ratings from 0% to 100% based on the severity of the disability. Percentages are assigned in increments of 10 (38 C.F.R. §§4.1-4.31).

[12] For example, veterans who may have been exposed to Agent Orange during the Vietnam War or veterans who may have diseases potentially related to service in the Gulf War may be eligible to receive care.

[13] Veterans with no service-connected conditions and who are Medicaid eligible, or who have an income below a certain VA means-test threshold and below a median income threshold for the geographic area in which they live, are also eligible to enroll in the VA health care system.

[14] The Veterans Programs Enhancement Act of 1998 (P.L. 105-368) gave veterans returning from combat operations a special two-year period of eligibility for health care from the VA without having to satisfy a means test or to demonstrate a service-connected disability. The National Defense Authorization Act (NDAA), FY2008 (P.L. 110-181) extended the period of enrollment for VA health care from two to five years for veterans who served in a theater of combat operations after November 11, 1998 (generally, Operation Enduring Freedom (OEF), Operation Iraqi Freedom (OIF), and Operation New Dawn (OND) veterans).

[15] All enrolled veterans are offered a standard medical benefits package, which is described in detail in 38 C.F.R. §17.38 (2011).

[16] TRICARE provides medical care to active duty servicemembers and other eligible beneficiaries (such as military retirees) through a combination of direct care in military clinics and hospitals and civilian-purchased care. For more information on TRICARE see, CRS Report RL33537, Military Medical Care: Questions and Answers, by Don J. Jansen.

[17] 38 U.S.C. §1729. Veterans who are rated as 50% or more service-connected disabled are exempt from all copayments. The VA is also required to collect reasonable charges for medical care or services (including prescription drugs) from a third-party insurer if the care provided would be covered under a private insurance plan; however, the VA does not collect reimbursements from Medicare or Medicaid. 38 U.S.C. §1729(a)(2)(D); 38 C.F.R. §17.101(a)(1)(i) (2011).

[18] In general, an appropriations act makes budget authority available beginning on October 1 of the fiscal year for which the appropriations act is passed ("budget year"). However, there are some types of appropriations that do not follow this pattern; among them are advance appropriations. An advance appropriation means appropriation of new budget authority that becomes available one or more fiscal years beyond the fiscal year for which the appropriations act was passed (i.e., beyond the budget year).

[19] Codified at 38 U.S.C. §117.

[20] Mandatory programs funded through the annual appropriations process are commonly referred to as appropriated entitlements. In general, appropriators have little control over the amounts provided for appropriated entitlements; rather, the authorizing statute establishes the program parameters (e.g., eligibility rules, benefit levels) that entitle certain recipients to payments. If Congress does not appropriate the money necessary to meet these commitments, entitled recipients (e.g., individuals, states, or other entities) may have legal recourse. For an overview of mandatory spending see, CRS Report RL33074, Mandatory Spending Since 1962, by D. Andrew Austin and Mindy R. Levit.

[21] Funding for discretionary programs are provided and controlled through the annual appropriations process. For more information see, CRS Report R41726, Discretionary Budget Authority by Subfunction: An Overview, by D. Andrew Austin.

[22] Department of Veterans Affairs, FY2013 Budget Submission, Summary Volume, Volume 1 of 4, February 2012, p. 2B-2.

[23] A major part of this discussion was drawn from U.S. Government Accountability Office, Veterans' Health Care: VA Uses a Projection Model to Develop Most of Its Health Care Budget Estimate to Inform the President's Budget Request, GAO-11-205, January 2011, pp. 4-8.

[24] The Veterans' Health Care Eligibility Reform Act of 1996 (P.L. 104-262) required the VHA to manage the provision of hospital care and medical services through an enrollment system based on a system of priorities.

[25] Department of Veterans Affairs, FY2013 Budget Submission, Medical Programs and Information Technology Programs, Volume 2 of 4, February 2012, p. 1A-6.

[26] VHA uses methodologies other than the EHCPM to develop estimates of the amount of resources needed for longterm care services, and various legislative and health care related initiatives that may change from year to year.

[27] U.S. Congress, Conference Committees, Consolidated Appropriations Act, 2004, conference report to accompany H.R. 2673, 108th Cong., 1st sess., H.Rept. 108-401, p. 1036.

[28] In its FY2008 budget request to Congress, the VA requested the transfer of food service operations costs from the medical facilities appropriations to the medical services appropriations. The House and Senate Appropriations Committees concurred with this request. The cost of food service operations support hospital food service workers, provisions, and supplies related to the direct care of patients.

[29] Biomedical engineering services include the maintenance and repair of all medical equipment used in the treatment, monitoring, diagnosis, or therapy of patients.

[30] For more information on CBOCs, see CRS Report R41044, Veterans Health Administration: Community-Based Outpatient Clinics, by Sidath Viranga Panangala.

[31] Vet Centers are community-based counseling centers, that provide a wide range of social and psychological services such as professional readjustment counseling to veterans who have served in a combat zone, military sexual trauma (MST) counseling, bereavement counseling for families who experience an active duty death, substance abuse assessments and referral,

medical referral, veterans' benefits explanation and referral, and employment counseling, among other services.

[32] VISN offices provide management and oversight to the medical centers and clinics within their assigned geographic areas. Each VISN office is responsible for allocating funds to facilities, clinics, and programs within its region and coordinating the delivery of health care to veterans.

[33] 38 U.S.C. §7303(a)(3). The Office of Research and Development (ORD) within the Veterans Health Administration (VHA) manages the medical research program. The medical research program encompasses, among other things, biomedical laboratory research, clinical trials, health services research, and rehabilitation research.

[34] The Consolidated Omnibus Budget Reconciliation Act of 1985 (P.L. 99-272), enacted into law in 1986 established means testing for veterans seeking care for nonservice-connected conditions. The Balanced Budget Act of 1997 (P.L. 105-33) established the Department of Veterans Affairs Medical Care Collections Fund (MCCF) gave the VHA the authority to retain these funds in the MCCF. Instead of returning the funds to the Treasury, the VA can use them, without fiscal year limitations, for medical services for veterans. In FY2004, the Administration's budget requested consolidating several existing medical collections accounts into one MCCF. The conferees of the Consolidated Appropriations Act of 2004 (H.Rept. 108-401) recommended that collections that would otherwise be deposited in the Health Services Improvement Fund (former name), Veterans Extended Care Revolving Fund (former name), Special Therapeutic and Rehabilitation Activities Fund (former name), Medical Facilities Revolving Fund (former name), and the Parking Revolving Fund (former name) should be deposited in MCCF. The Consolidated Appropriations Act of 2005 (P.L. 108-447, H.Rept. 108-792) provided the VA with permanent authority to deposit funds from these five accounts into the MCCF.

[35] Department of Veterans Affairs, FY2013 Budget Submission, Medical Programs and Information Technology Programs, Volume 2 of 4, February 2012, p 1C-18.

[36] Ibid.

[37] U.S. Congress, House Committee on Veterans' Affairs, U.S. Department of Veterans Affairs Budget Request for Fiscal Year 2012, 112th Cong., 1st sess., February 17, 2011 (Washington: GPO, 2011), p. 163. VHA is statutorily [42 U.S.C §1395f(c)] prohibited from receiving Medicare payments for services provided to Medicare-covered veterans.

[38] For a detailed description of the FY2012 VHA appropriations see, CRS Report R41944, Veterans' Medical Care: FY2012 Appropriations, by Sidath Viranga Panangala.

[39] In August 2010, VA issued regulations establishing presumptive service connection for three new conditions: B-cell leukemias, such as hairy cell leukemia; Parkinson's disease; and ischemic heart disease (see Department of Veterans Affairs, "Diseases Associated With Exposure to Certain Herbicide Agents (Hairy Cell Leukemia and Other Chronic B-Cell Leukemias, Parkinson's Disease and Ischemic Heart Disease)," 75 Federal Register 53202-53216, August 31, 2010). This rule change resulted in an increase in service-connected patients, and added new patients to VA's health care system. Furthermore, it changed the priority levels of veterans currently enrolled in VA's health care system.

[40] In 2008, the VA, through regulation, established a presumptive service connection for ALS, making those veterans with ALS eligible for free health care for symptoms associated with ALS (see Department of Veterans Affairs, "Presumption of Service Connection for Amyotrophic Lateral Sclerosis," 73 Federal Register 54691-54693, September 23, 2008). To be eligible for this presumptive service connection, a veteran must have served on continuous active duty for a period of 90 days or more. For more information on

presumptive service connection see CRS Report R41405, Veterans Affairs: Presumptive Service Connection and Disability Compensation, coordinated by Sidath Viranga Panangala. U.S. Department of Veterans Affairs, FY2013 Budget Submission, Medical Programs and Information Technology Programs, Volume 2 of 4, February 2012, p. 1A-3.

[41] Letter from Steven D. Aitken, Deputy General Counsel Office of Management and Budget (OMB), to Julia C. Matta, Assistant General Counsel for Appropriations and Budget, U.S. Government Accountability Office, April 23, 2012. http://www.murray.senate.gov/public/_cache/files/f8868d52-eec0-43a5-b5c8-cecbff4596e/VASequesterQuestion.pdf.

[42] U.S. Congress, House Committee on the Budget, Concurrent Resolution On The Budget—Fiscal Year 2013, Report to accompany H.Con.Res. 112, 112th Cong., 2nd sess., March 23, 2012, H.Rept. 112-421 (Washington: GPO, 2012), p. 107.

[43] U.S. Congress, House Committee on Appropriations, Military Construction and Veterans Affairs and Related Agencies Appropriations bill 2013, report to accompany H.R. 5854, 112th Cong., 2nd sess., May 23, 2010, p. 35.

[44] Ibid., p. 36.

[45] "Military Construction and Veterans Affairs and Related Agencies Appropriations Act, 2013," Consideration of the bill (H.R. 5854) making appropriations for military construction, the Department of Veterans Affairs, and related agencies for the fiscal year ending September 30, 2013, and for other purposes, Congressional Record, vol. 158 (May 31, 2012), p. H3328. The Veterans' Mental Health and Other Care Improvements Act of 2008 (P.L. 110-387), was signed into law on October 10, 2008. Section 403 of this law required VA to conduct a pilot programs during a three-year period to provide non-VA health care services through contractual arrangements to eligible veterans. Project ARCH is the name of this pilot program.

[46] Ibid., p. H3327.

[47] U.S. Congress, Senate Committee on Appropriations, Military Construction and Veterans Affairs, and Related Agencies Appropriations bill, 2013, report to accompany S. 3215, 112th Cong., 2nd sess., May 22, 2012, p. 42.

[48] Ibid., p. 48.

[49] U.S. Congress, House Committee on Veterans' Affairs, Subcommittee on Health, Legislative Hearing on H.R.4241, 111th Cong., 2nd sess., March 3, 2010 (Washington: GPO, 2010), pp. 22-23.

In: Veteran's Health Care
Editor: Claude Da Costa

ISBN: 978-1-62417-371-4

Chapter 7

VETERANS' HEALTH CARE BUDGET: BETTER LABELING OF SERVICES AND MORE DETAILED INFORMATION COULD IMPROVE THE CONGRESSIONAL BUDGET JUSTIFICATION*

United States Government Accountability Office

ABBREVIATIONS

CBJ	Congressional Budget Justification
CHAMPVA	Civilian Health and Medical Program of the Department of Veterans Affairs
CWVV	Children of Women Vietnam Veterans
EHCPM	Enrollee Health Care Projection Model
FMP	Foreign Medical Program
OMB	Office of Management and Budget
VA	Department of Veterans Affairs
VA CLC	Veterans Affairs Community Living Centers
VHA	Veterans Health Administration

* This is an edited, reformatted and augmented version of The United States Government Accountability Office publication, Report to Congressional Committees, GAO-12-908, dated September 2012.

WHY GAO DID THIS STUDY

The VA operates one of the largest health care delivery systems in the nation. Within VA, VHA provides a range of health care services for eligible veterans, such as primary care, inpatient and outpatient surgery, and nursing home care. In the past, VHA received medical care funds primarily through a single appropriations account. However, to "provide better oversight and receive a more accurate accounting of funds," in 2004, Congress established a new three appropriations account structure.

GAO was asked to (1) describe the relationship between VHA's appropriations account structure and VA's development of the budget request; and (2) examine how VA presents information about the three VHA appropriations accounts in its CBJ. To conduct this work GAO reviewed VA budget policy documents, VA's fiscal year 2009-2013 CBJs, prior GAO work on budget formulation at VA, and interviewed VHA budget officials.

WHAT GAO RECOMMENDS

GAO recommends that VA label health care services consistently so it is clear what services are being referred to across appropriations accounts. GAO also recommends that VA further consult with congressional decision makers when determining what detailed information related to appropriations accounts should be presented—and how— in its CBJ. VA generally agrees with GAO's conclusions and concurs with GAO's recommendations. VA stated what actions it will take to implement the recommendations.

WHAT GAO FOUND

The Department of Veterans Affairs (VA) creates its budget request through its Enrollee Health Care Projection Model (EHCPM) using data from systems designed for the former single-account structure. These systems do not explicitly consider the three appropriations accounts: Medical Services, Medical Support and Compliance, and Medical Facilities. According to Veterans Health Administration (VHA) officials, VHA formulates its budget based on the single appropriations account, in part, because the systems to formulate the request were in place prior to 2004, which was when the three-account structure was established. VA then presents the information in the Congressional Budget Justification (CBJ) by taking the data developed by the EHCPM and then, based on historical percentages and future projections, assigning the requested amounts to the three appropriations accounts.

The information about VA's health care accounts in its CBJ can be difficult to follow because information is not displayed consistently across the three medical care appropriations accounts. This is due to inconsistent labeling and varying levels of detail among the three appropriations accounts throughout the justification. VHA officials stated that inconsistent labeling in the CBJ's tables was inadvertent. With respect to varying levels of detail among the three appropriations accounts, VHA officials said that the administrative and facilities costs for some programs are relatively small compared to the Medical Services costs. Thus they are not displayed for all three accounts. However, in at least one instance, the amount of administrative and facilities costs not shown was about 31 percent—a total of $1.05 billion—of the program's cost. Finally, VA presents several summary tables that highlight program costs; however, information on how most of these costs break down across the three accounts cannot be found in the CBJ. The lack of such account-level information can make it more difficult for congressional decision makers to make appropriations decisions and to conduct oversight.

September 18, 2012

The Honorable Patty Murray
Chairman

The Honorable Richard Burr
Ranking Member
Committee on Veterans' Affairs United States Senate

The Honorable Jeff Miller
Chairman

The Honorable Bob Filner
Ranking Member
Committee on Veterans' Affairs
House of Representatives

The Department of Veterans Affairs (VA) operates one of the largest health care delivery systems in the nation. Within VA, the Veterans Health Administration (VHA) provides a range of health care services for eligible veterans, including primary care, inpatient and outpatient surgery, prosthetics, mental health services, prescription drugs, and nursing home care. In the past, VHA received medical care funds primarily through a single appropriations account.

However, in 2004, Congress established a new account structure to "provide better oversight and receive a more accurate accounting of funds."[1] This changed VHA's medical care appropriations account structure from one account to three: Medical Services, Medical Support and Compliance, and Medical Facilities. These three accounts are considered to comprise VHA's "medical care" accounts.

An appropriations account structure broadly reflects how the House and Senate appropriations committees make resource allocation choices, the preferences of these appropriations committees, and the types of control and incentives these committees consider most important. Previously, we reported that changes to the budget structure and Congressional Budget Justifications (CBJ)—documents that support agency budget requests—have the potential to help reframe budget choices.[2]

Moreover, in the past, we have emphasized the importance of transparency in federal agencies' CBJs—that is, they should be clear and easy to understand—in part because Congress relies on the information in them to make resource allocation decisions and conduct oversight.[3] This report responds to your request that we (1) describe the relationship between VHA's appropriations account structure and VA's development of the budget request and (2) examine how VA presents information about the three VHA appropriations accounts in its CBJ.

To complete our work, we reviewed VA budget policy documents, its fiscal years 2009 through 2013 CBJs, and our prior work on budget formulation at VA, and we interviewed VHA budget officials. We conducted this performance audit from June 2011 to September 2012 in accordance with generally accepted government auditing standards. Those standards require that we plan and perform the audit to obtain sufficient, appropriate evidence to provide a reasonable basis for our findings and conclusions based on our audit objectives.

We believe that the evidence obtained provides a reasonable basis for our findings and conclusions based on our audit objectives.

BACKGROUND

In fiscal year 2011, approximately 6.2 million patients received health care from VA.[4] In providing that care, VA operates 152 hospitals, 133 nursing homes, 824 community-based outpatient clinics, and other facilities through 21 regional health care networks.

A variety of activities are funded through VHA's three appropriations accounts for medical care:

- The *Medical Services* account includes funds for health care services provided to eligible veterans and beneficiaries in VA's medical centers, outpatient clinic facilities, contract hospitals, state homes, and outpatient programs on a fee basis.[5] For fiscal year 2012, VA received more than $39.6 billion in the Medical Services account.[6]
- The *Medical Support and Compliance* account includes funds for the management and administration of the VA health care system, including financial management, human resources, and logistics. For fiscal year 2012, VA received more than $5.5 billion in the Medical Support and Compliance account.[7]
- The *Medical Facilities* account includes funds for the operation and maintenance of the VA health care system's capital infrastructure, such as costs associated with nonrecurring maintenance, utilities, facility repair, laundry services, and grounds keeping.[8] For fiscal year 2012, VA received more than $5.4 billion in the Medical Facilities account.[9]

The amount of funding Congress gives VA to provide its health care services is determined by the annual appropriations process. The development of VA's annual budget estimate is inherently complex, as assumptions and imperfect information are used to project the likely quantity and cost of the health care services VHA expects it will be required to provide.10 Unlike most other agencies, VA receives advance appropriations for health care in addition to annual appropriations.[11] Accordingly, in preparation for the appropriations process, VA begins developing an annual estimate of the resources needed to provide its health care services for 2 fiscal years well in advance.[12] This budget estimate is reviewed through successively higher levels within the agency and revised until consolidated into a department-wide annual budget estimate that is submitted to the Office of Management and Budget (OMB) for review and consideration. OMB subsequently includes both an appropriations request for VA health care services for 1 fiscal year and an advance appropriations request for the next fiscal year in the President's annual budget request.[13] This estimate must include assumptions about future economic conditions, presidential policies, and congressional actions that may affect the funding needs in the year for which the request is made. Because VA is required to provide services to eligible veterans, VA's budget estimates must also accommodate the future demand for the total cost of providing health care services, including direct patient costs as well as costs associated with management, administration, and maintenance of facilities.

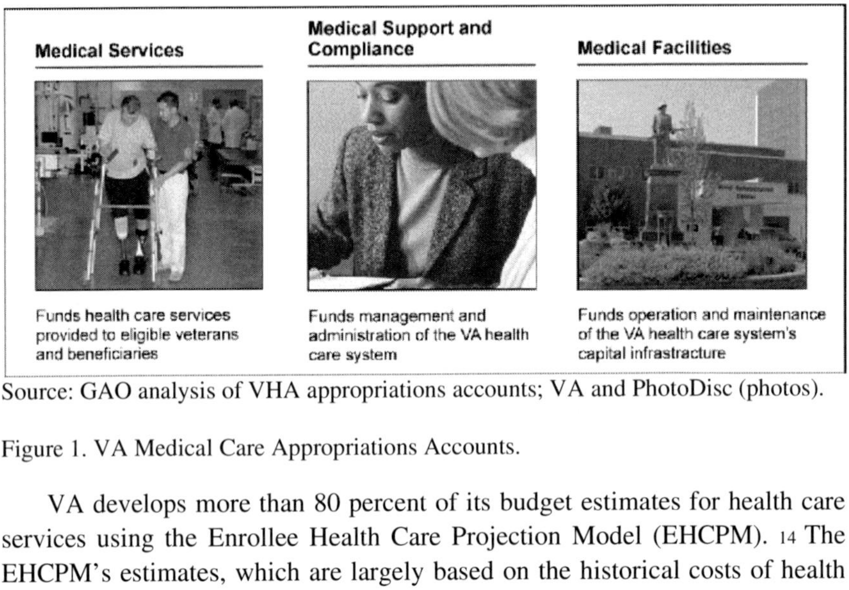

Source: GAO analysis of VHA appropriations accounts; VA and PhotoDisc (photos).

Figure 1. VA Medical Care Appropriations Accounts.

VA develops more than 80 percent of its budget estimates for health care services using the Enrollee Health Care Projection Model (EHCPM). [14] The EHCPM's estimates, which are largely based on the historical costs of health care services, include three basic components: the projected number of veterans who will be enrolled in VA health care, the projected demand for health care services by these enrollees, and the projected unit cost of providing these services. VHA uses the EHCPM to estimate the resources needed to meet expected demand for over 70 health care services such as surgery, pharmacy, and prosthetics. Other methods are used to develop the remaining parts of its budget request; that is, the costs of long-term care and other health care programs.[15] According to VA, starting in the President's fiscal year 2014 budget request, long-term care estimates will be developed using a new model similar to and grounded in the EHCPM, but specific to the nature of long-term care costs. In support of the President's budget request, VA prepares a CBJ.

This CBJ provides Congress with estimates and other information that support the policies and spending decisions represented in the President's budget request, including information on what VA plans to achieve with the resources requested. In particular, the CBJ reflects detailed information on estimates of funding needed for ongoing health care services and health care-related initiatives proposed by the Secretary of VA and the President and provides information about agency priorities, as well as the implications of the requested amounts for VHA's provision of health care services to veterans. While VA must present the budget using the three- account structure, as mentioned previously, it also presents the three accounts in aggregate under the name "medical care." Instead of breaking down obligations by account, the medical care table breaks down obligations using other broad health care categories such as rehabilitative care, mental health, and institutional long-term care.

The CBJ is a key document that helps Congress make appropriations decisions, conduct oversight, and provide control over VA's funds. The structure of the CBJ reflects OMB guidance and the interests of the House and Senate appropriations committees. This allows agencies the flexibility to tailor the contents of the CBJ to the various needs of the primary users of this information; that is, the appropriations committees of jurisdiction. Over time, the content and structure of CBJs have evolved to accommodate changing circumstances and priorities. According to VA officials, the CBJ was developed by VHA along with OMB in response to the appropriations committee's questions about specific areas of medical care.

VA's Budget Request Is Based on Data from Systems Designed for the Former Single-Account Structure

VA creates its budget request through the EHCPM using data from systems designed for the former single-account structure.[16] These systems do not explicitly consider the three appropriations accounts.[17] According to VHA officials, VHA formulates its budget based on the single appropriations account, in part, because the systems to formulate the request were in place prior to 2004, which was when the three-account structure was established.

VA presents the budget request in the CBJ using the three-account structure created by Congress. According to VHA officials, this is done by taking the data about the costs of the over 70 health care services developed by the EHCPM and then based on historical percentages and future projections, assigning the requested amounts to the three appropriations accounts.

VA Provides Inconsistent Information across VHA's Three Medical Care Appropriations Accounts

VA's CBJ can be difficult to follow because information is not displayed consistently across the three medical care appropriations accounts. There are three key reasons for this:

1. health care service labels are inconsistent across the three appropriations accounts,
2. health care services are described in varying levels of detail across the three appropriations accounts, and
3. summary tables lack detailed account-level information.

Consistent information across the three accounts is important to achieving the stated purposes of changing to the three-account structure; that is, to provide better oversight and a more accurate accounting of funds. Moreover, our past work states that in order to facilitate decision making, information needs to be clear and organized in a way that is meaningful to its users.[18] While the House and Senate appropriations committees are the primary users of the CBJ, other committees also use the information presented in the CBJ. For instance, the House and Senate Committees on Veterans' Affairs—the authorizing committees— use the CBJ as one tool in conducting oversight.

Health Care Service Labels Are Inconsistent across the Three Appropriations Accounts

Inconsistent service labels in the CBJ contribute to a confusing presentation. Service labels are inconsistent in that different labels may refer to the same services. For example, as shown in table 1, what is referred to as "psychiatric care" in the detailed presentation of the Medical Support and Compliance and Medical Facilities accounts is referred to as "mental health" in the detailed presentation for the Medical Services account.[19] We determined that mental health and psychiatric care refer to the same services by comparing the totals and confirming this with VHA officials. The situation is the same as with the Civilian Health and Medical Program of the Department of Veterans Affairs (CHAMPVA) in the Medical Support and Compliance and Medical Facilities accounts. As seen in table 1, this service is labeled as CHAMPVA, Spina Bifida, Foreign Medical Program (FMP), and Children of Women Vietnam Veterans (CWVV) in the displays of the Medical Services account. The smaller programs of Spina Bifida, FMP, and CWVV are included in the Medical Support and Compliance and Medical Facilities accounts, but not listed by name. According to VHA officials, the inconsistent labeling was inadvertent.

Table 1. Excerpts from VA's CBJ Showing Different Labels for the Same Service

Dollars in millions

				VHA medical care accounts		
Medical Support and Compliance		Medical Facilities		Medical Services		Total medical care
Description	2011 obligations	Description	2011 obligations	Description	2011 obligations	2011 obligations
Psychiatric care	$708	Psychiatric care	$827	Mental health	$3,984	$5,519
CHAMPVA	78	CHAMPVA	5	CHAMPVA, Spina Bifida, FMP, and CWVV	1,138	1,221

Source: GAO presentation of VA's 2013 CBJ data.

Note: We created this table using data provided in the Department of Veterans Affairs Congressional Submission, FY 2013 Funding and FY 2014 Advance Appropriations Request, Vol. 2, Medical Programs and Information Technology Programs, 1A-5,1C-3, 1D-8, and 1E-12.

In addition to the inconsistencies in labeling among the same services, similar labeling may refer to entirely different services. For example, as shown in table 2, a user might think that the "acute hospital care" and "subacute care" services listed under the Medical Support and Compliance and Medical Facilities accounts are subcomponents of the "acute care" services shown under the Medical Services account. However, they are not subcomponents of acute care. The terminology and presentation are not consistent with terminology and presentation used elsewhere. According to VHA officials, the tables represent several ways of breaking down the subcomponents of the total appropriation and are a response to requests for different ways to display the information that have been requested over time.

Table 2. Excerpts from VA's CBJ Showing Similar Labels for Different Services

VHA medical care accounts						
Medical Support and Compliance		Medical Facilities		Medical Services		Total medical care
Description	2011 obligations	Description	2011 obligations	Description	2011 obligations	2011 obligations
			Acute care		$27,049	$34,933
Acute hospital care	$1,130	Acute hospital care	$1,296			
Subacute care	10	Subacute care	12			

Source: GAO presentation of VA's 2013 CBJ data.

Note: We created this table using data provided in the Department of Veterans Affairs Congressional Submission, FY 2013 Funding and FY 2014 Advance Appropriations Request, Vol.2, Medical Programs and Information Technology Programs, 1A-5, 1C-3, 1D-8, and 1E-12.

Levels of Detail Vary Across the Three Appropriations Accounts

Another area of inconsistency in the CBJ is that levels of detail vary across the three appropriations accounts. Specifically, the level of detail provided for the Medical Services account is significantly greater than what is provided for the Medical Support and Compliance and Medical Facilities accounts.

For example, as shown in table 3, resources requested for VA community living centers (VA CLC), community nursing homes, and state nursing homes are provided for the Medical Services account but not for the Medical Support and Compliance or Medical Facilities accounts.

While the state nursing home, community nursing homes, and VA CLC programs do consume resources from the Medical Support and Compliance and Medical Facilities accounts, the amounts from those accounts are not shown.

Table 3. Information from VA's CBJ Comparing Obligations Provided for Nursing Home Care and Long-Term Care

Dollars in millions

		VHA medical care accounts					
Medical Support and Compliance		*Medical Facilities*		*Medical Services*		*Total medical care*	
Description	*2011 obligations*	*Description*	*2011 obligations*	*Description*	*2011 obligations*	*2011 obligations*	*Difference–(not Shown in CBJ)*[b]
Nursing home care	$481	Nursing home care	$578	Nursing home care[a]	$3,756	$4,815	$1,059
				VA CLC	2,374	3,425	1,051
				Community nursing homes	607	614	7
				State nursing homes	775	775	0

Source: GAO presentation of VA's 2013 CBJ data.

Note: We created this table using data provided in the Department of Veterans Affairs Congressional Submission, FY 2013 Funding and FY 2014 Advance Appropriations Request, Vol. 2, Medical Programs and Information Technology Programs, 1A-5,1C-3, 1C-24, 1D-8, and 1E-12.

[a] While nursing home care does not appear in aggregate alongside its subcomponents in the CBJ, for the sake of clarity, we present this information together in this table.

[b] This represents the difference between the dollar amounts provided in the medical care detailed table and the medical services detailed table.

VHA officials explained that they do not produce separate estimates or display obligations for the Medical Support and Compliance and Medical Facilities costs because the costs for those accounts are relatively small compared to the Medical Services account. However, in at least one instance, the amount not shown was considerable.

For example, about 31 percent—a total of $1.05 billion—was obligated for administrative and facilities costs combined for VA CLC, but the CBJ does not show this number or the specific breakdown between the Medical Support and Compliance and Medical Facilities accounts.

Congress may consider the administrative and facilities costs for VA CLC to be significant and important to decision making.

Summary Tables Detail Costs by Program but Not by Appropriations Accounts

VA presents several summary tables that highlight program costs; however, information on how most of these costs break down across the three accounts cannot be found in the CBJ. For example, in the table of "selected program highlights," which VA officials informed us is one of the key tables of interest to Congress, most program costs are not also broken out across the three accounts.[20] The lack of such account-level information can make it more difficult for Congressional decision makers to conduct oversight.

Congressional committees have recently requested more information about VA's spending and voiced concerns about VA's CBJ. Specifically, the House Committee on Appropriations recently requested that VA provide additional detail on, for example, administrative costs by headquarters, regional network, and medical center, in order to help inform congressional decisions.[21]

The Senate Committee on Appropriations also recently expressed concern that the "justifications continue to lack specificity and the degree of detail needed to ensure informed and timely evaluation of requested funds and proper oversight of a Department the size of the VA."[22] In addition, according to some authorizing committee staff, the CBJ is confusing and after the switch to the three-account structure, information in the CBJ has not become more detailed or transparent. According to VHA officials, the CBJ reflects the information Congress has asked VA to provide. They added that both the House and Senate appropriations committees have expressed an interest in more detailed information in the CBJ to increase oversight, but have not asked VA to change the structure or content of the CBJ as a whole.

CONCLUSION

VA's CBJ is intended to provide congressional committees with information they need to make decisions. To facilitate decision making, information needs to be clear and organized in a way that is meaningful to its users. Our work has demonstrated that there are concerns with the clarity and usefulness of the information presented in the CBJ. Users of the CBJ should be able to rely on consistency in labeling to help them understand the information being presented.

Increasing congressional oversight was one of the motivations to establish the current account structure. Our work has identified areas where the information as presented across the three accounts does not provide the level of detail desired to improve oversight. Various congressional committees have also stated that the information is not meeting their needs.

Recommendations for Executive Action

To improve the clarity and usefulness of information presented in VA's congressional budget justifications that support the President's budget request for VA health care, we recommend the Secretary of Veterans Affairs take the following two actions:

- Label health care services consistently so it is clear what services, such as mental health, are being referred to across appropriations accounts.
- Further consult with congressional decision makers to determine what detailed information related to the three appropriations accounts should be presented, and how, in its congressional budget justification.

Agency Comments

We provided a draft of this report to the Secretary of Veterans Affairs for comment. In its written comments his Chief of Staff generally agrees with our conclusions and concurs with our recommendations. In response to our first recommendation, VA stated they will undertake a review of the programmatic reference in the CBJ volume for the medical programs and standardize throughout.

In addition, VA will initiate discussions with the Office of Management and Budget to determine whether the references in the President's Budget Appendix can also be made consistent.

In response to our second recommendation, VA also stated it would consult with Congress to identify any additional information to include in the budget justification document.

Finally, VA provided technical comments that were incorporated, as appropriate.

Melissa Emrey-Arras
Acting Director
Strategic Issues

End Notes

[1] H.R. Rep. No. 108-401, at 1036 (2003).

[2] GAO, Performance Budgeting: Efforts to Restructure Budgets to Better Align Resources with Performance, GAO-05-117SP (Washington, D.C.: February 2005).

[3] GAO, Internal Revenue Service: Assessment of Budget Justification for Fiscal Year 2011 Identified Opportunities to Enhance Transparency, GAO-10-687R (Washington, D.C.: May 26, 2010).

[4] Eligibility is determined on the basis of service-connected disability, income, and other special statuses, such as former prisoners of war, and is used to determine priority for VA services. VA is required to provide a specified set of health care services, including hospital care, to eligible veterans. 38 U.S.C. §§ 1710(a)(1), (2), 1701(5), (6). VA is authorized to provide these health care services to other veterans not identified in these groups. 38 U.S.C.§ 1710(a)(3). The population of veterans to whom VA is required to provide nursing home care is more limited than the population to whom VA is required to provide other health care services, although VA also makes nursing home care available to other veterans on a discretionary basis as resources permit. See 38 U.S.C. § 1710A.

[5] Beneficiaries may include nonveterans, such as family members receiving Civilian Health and Medical Program of the Department of Veterans Affairs benefits.

[6] Pub. L. No. 112-10, div. B, title X, § 2015, 125 Stat. 38, 175 (Apr. 15, 2011). In addition to new appropriations that VA receives during the annual appropriations process, funding may also be available from unobligated balances of multiyear appropriations, which remain available for a fixed period of time in excess of 1 fiscal year. For example, VA's fiscal year 2011 appropriations provided that $1.2 billion be available for 2 fiscal years. Pub. L. No. 112-10, § 2014. VA's other sources of funding include collections and reimbursements. VA's collections include third-party payments from veterans' private health care insurance for the treatment of non-service-connected conditions and veterans' copayments for outpatient medications. VA's reimbursements include amounts VA receives for services provided under service agreements with the Department of Defense. See GAO, Veterans' Health Care Budget: Transparency and Reliability of Some Estimates Supporting President's Request Could Be Improved, GAO-12-689 (Washington, D.C.: June 11, 2012).

[7] Pub. L. No. 112-10, § 2015.

[8] This account does not include funding for major or minor construction or for information technology because separate appropriations provide funds for these purposes.

[9] Pub. L. No. 112-10, § 2015.

[10] GAO, VA Health Care: Challenges in Budget Formulation and Execution, GAO-09-459T (Washington, D.C.: Mar. 12, 2009).

[11] The Veterans Health Care Budget Reform and Transparency Act of 2009 provided that VA's annual appropriations for health care also include advance appropriations that become available 1 fiscal year after the fiscal year for which the appropriations act was enacted. Pub. L. No. 111-81, § 3, 123 Stat. 2137, 2137–38 (2009), codified at 38 U.S.C. § 117. The act provided for advance appropriations for VA's Medical Services, Medical Support and Compliance, and Medical Facilities appropriations accounts. The act also required VA to include additional information in its annual CBJ. Specifically, the VA Secretary must include detailed estimates of the funds necessary to provide VA health care services for the fiscal year for which advance appropriations will be provided.

[12] VA begins formulating a budget request approximately 10 months before the President submits the budget to Congress in early February. This is approximately 18 months before the start of the fiscal year to which the request relates and about 30 months prior to the start of the fiscal year to which the advance appropriations request relates.

[13] For example, in the spring of 2011, VA began formulating the President's VA health care request for fiscal year 2013 and an advance appropriations request for fiscal year 2014. In the spring of 2012, VA began updating the request for fiscal year 2014. Before or during fiscal year 2013, Congress and the President may enact advance appropriations for the needs of fiscal year 2014. If Congress and the President later enact different appropriations for fiscal year 2014, those appropriations would then supersede any previously enacted advance appropriations.

[14] GAO-11-205.

[15] The estimates for these services are based on factors, such as recent data on the costs and the amount of care VHA provided to veterans, VHA's policy goals for providing such services, and projections of the number of users.

[16] The Decision Support System is VHA's cost accounting system, which aggregates cost information from VA's workload and financial systems. This system provides EHCPM with data to develop future year budget estimates.

[17] Although the systems used to formulate VA's budget request in the CBJ do not explicitly consider the three appropriations accounts, VHA officials told us that they manage their resources within the appropriation limits.

[18] GAO-10-687R and GAO-05-117SP.

[19] The CBJ presents two levels of detail for the Medical Services account. Although the detailed presentation uses different labels than what is shown for the other two accounts, the less detailed presentation provides the same labels across all three accounts.

[20] One exception to this is information on CHAMPVA/FMP/Spina Bifida/CWVV. Account-level information on this program is found in CBJ Vol. 2, Medical Programs and Information Technology Programs, 1A-5,1C-3, 1D-8, and 1E-12.

[21] H.R. Rep. No. 112-491, at 47 (2012). 22S. Rep. No. 112-168, at 32 (2012).

INDEX

#

9/11, 37

A

access, 3, 10, 16, 95
accounting, xiii, 66, 95, 124, 126, 130
accreditation, 87
adverse event, ix, x, 52, 53, 54, 55, 56, 57, 58, 59, 60, 61
Afghanistan, 8, 110
age, 45, 46, 49
agencies, 12, 76, 93, 97, 122, 126, 127, 129
Air Force, ix, 32, 33, 37, 38
Alaska, 28
Alaska Natives, 28
ALS, 105, 121
appropriations, vii, xii, xiii, 4, 28, 49, 85, 90, 91, 92, 95, 97, 100, 104, 105, 106, 107, 108, 109, 111, 114, 120, 121, 122, 124, 125, 126, 127, 128, 129, 130, 132, 134, 135, 136, 137
Appropriations Act, 92, 95, 100, 101, 102, 104, 121, 122
Appropriations Committee, xii, 90, 106, 107, 109, 112, 115, 120
armed forces, 119
assessment, 54, 68, 78, 84, 87
assessment tools, 78
assets, 29
audit(s), xi, 53, 68, 84, 86, 126
authority(s), viii, xi, 2, 4, 20, 59, 61, 90, 92, 93, 94, 97, 99, 104, 105, 106, 107, 112, 114, 120, 121
awareness, 60

B

bed-wetting, 47
beneficiaries, 10, 28, 42, 43, 44, 46, 48, 119, 127
benefits, vii, viii, ix, xi, 2, 6, 9, 10, 23, 25, 26, 27, 31, 32, 33, 34, 35, 36, 37, 38, 42, 45, 46, 47, 68, 89, 90, 93, 94, 117, 118, 119, 121, 136
blood, 77
bone, 47
bone marrow, 47
bone marrow transplant, 47
bowel, 15
brain, 13
breakdown, 93, 133
budget allocation, 93
Budget Committee, 107
budget resolution, 105, 107
budgetary resources, 93

C

cardiac surgery, 12
caregivers, viii, 1, 96
cash, viii, 31, 32, 99
cataract, 13
category a, 25, 42
certificate, 12
certification, 11, 33
challenges, 73
Chief of Staff, 135
children, 29, 42
chronic illness, 13
cities, 97
Civilian Health and Medical Program of the Department of Veterans Affairs (CHAMPVA), viii, ix, 1, 7, 41, 42, 49, 131
clarity, 65, 133, 134, 135
classes, 10
classification, 23, 117
cleaning, xi, 55, 64
clinical judgment, 15
clinical trials, 9, 97, 121
clothing, 78
Coast Guard, 33
cognitive impairment, 13
colleges, 97
commercial, 97
Committees on Appropriations, 97
commodity, 85, 88
community, 13, 14, 15, 21, 59, 96, 120, 127, 132
compensation, xi, 6, 11, 13, 21, 34, 38, 42, 59, 89, 90, 91, 93, 94, 99, 118
complexity, 37, 67, 82, 83, 85, 88
compliance, xi, xii, 60, 64, 65, 66, 68, 69, 76, 77, 78, 79, 80, 81, 82, 83, 84, 86, 87, 90, 92, 95, 99, 104, 105, 107, 109, 111, 114
conference, 100, 120
Congress, x, xi, xiii, 1, 4, 7, 20, 22, 26, 27, 28, 31, 36, 41, 42, 49, 52, 67, 89, 92, 93, 95, 97, 98, 99, 100, 105, 106, 108, 120, 121, 122, 124, 126, 127, 129, 133, 134, 135, 137
congressional budget, 135
Consolidated Appropriations Act, 92, 100, 104, 111, 114, 120, 121
construction, 14, 93, 94, 95, 96, 99, 122, 136
contamination, 77
contingency, 99, 100
copayments for medical services, viii, 2, 17
cost, 10, 14, 15, 18, 20, 42, 47, 48, 70, 77, 96, 97, 116, 120, 125, 127, 137
cost accounting, 137
counseling, viii, 2, 7, 9, 10, 17, 58, 110, 120
current account, 135

D

daily living, 12, 13, 15
database, 75
death rate, 44
decision makers, 124, 125, 134, 135
deficiencies, x, 13, 52, 57, 58, 61, 68, 84
deficit, 106
delegates, 87
dental care, viii, 2, 10, 12, 47, 68
Department of Defense, 38, 42, 92, 97, 104, 136
Department of Veterans Affairs (VA), vii, viii, xi, 1, 2, 31, 32, 41, 64, 66, 82, 89, 90, 111, 124, 126
diabetes, 13
dialysis, 77, 82
directives, x, 52, 60
directors, 58
disability, xi, 4, 5, 11, 13, 16, 17, 18, 20, 21, 22, 23, 24, 26, 27, 34, 38, 42, 44, 45, 49, 89, 90, 91, 93, 94, 116, 118, 119, 136
discharges, 34, 35
disclosure, 55, 59, 61
diseases, 13, 27, 29, 59, 67, 70, 73, 77, 80, 85, 86, 87, 119
disinfection, 86
disposition, 96
DME, 48

draft, xii, 58, 81, 90, 109, 135
drugs, 9, 13
due process, 57
durable medical equipment, viii, 2, 9, 47, 48

E

earnings, 29
education, ix, 15, 31, 32, 37, 83, 85, 88, 90, 91, 93, 94, 96, 118
eligibility criteria, ix, xi, 10, 16, 18, 28, 32, 89
e-mail, ix, 52, 58
emergency, viii, 2, 16, 18, 21, 28
employees, vii, 1, 2, 38, 59, 96
employment, x, 12, 21, 25, 38, 40, 52, 59, 61, 91, 93, 94, 99, 118, 121
employment status, 59
endoscopy, 82
engineering, 96, 120
enrollment, xi, 3, 4, 5, 6, 7, 16, 22, 24, 27, 28, 42, 48, 89, 91, 117, 119, 120
equipment, viii, xi, 2, 9, 47, 48, 55, 59, 63, 64, 66, 67, 71, 72, 73, 78, 82, 85, 86, 88, 96, 120
evidence, xi, 32, 33, 38, 53, 58, 68, 84, 126
examinations, ix, 47, 52
exclusion, 21, 47
expenditures, 42, 44
expertise, 55
exposure, 20, 23, 86, 117

F

families, viii, 31, 32, 45, 120
family members, 7, 44, 45, 136
FDA, 9
federal facilities, 18, 28
federal funds, 22
federal government, vii, 3, 85, 88
federal law, 54, 55, 57, 60
Federal Register, 27, 49, 121
female veterans, viii, 2, 10
fertilization, viii, 2, 9, 10
financial, viii, 6, 7, 17, 31, 32, 116, 127, 137
financial system, 137
fiscal year 2009, xiii, 124
flexibility, 116, 129
food, 96, 120
Food and Drug Administration, 9, 86
funding, xii, 28, 90, 92, 93, 96, 97, 105, 106, 108, 111, 114, 127, 129, 136
funds, xii, 29, 92, 95, 96, 99, 104, 108, 112, 115, 121, 124, 126, 127, 129, 130, 134, 136, 137

G

GAO, x, xi, xiii, 51, 54, 61, 63, 64, 65, 70, 83, 85, 86, 87, 88, 120, 123, 124, 128, 131, 132, 133, 136, 137
gender-specific care, viii, 2
Georgia, 82
GI Bill, ix, 32, 37
GI Bill Improvement Act, ix, 32, 37
glasses, 13
governor, 6
grants, 53, 91, 97, 119
guidance, x, 52, 53, 58, 60, 65, 74, 75, 79, 129
guidelines, 71, 75, 86, 92, 104, 112, 114
gynecological care, viii, 2, 10

H

hairy cell leukemia, 121
hazards, 3
head and neck cancer, 20
Health and Human Services, 21
health care costs, 97
health care programs, 93, 128
health care system, vii, ix, x, xi, 3, 7, 16, 17, 18, 20, 27, 41, 51, 52, 55, 66, 89, 91, 96, 97, 119, 121, 127
health condition, 33
health insurance, 7, 18, 19, 20, 21, 25, 46, 48, 91
health services, 9, 121

health status, 28
hearing impairment, 13
heart attack, 5, 6
heart disease, 121
hepatitis, 73, 77
HHS, 21
history, 21
HIV, 63, 70, 73, 77
home care services, 14
homes, 14, 15, 96, 116, 127, 132
hospice, 9, 47
host, 14
hostility, 23, 117
House, xii, 26, 27, 28, 42, 48, 51, 66, 90, 100, 101, 102, 104, 105, 107, 108, 109, 111, 112, 114, 115, 120, 121, 122, 125, 126, 129, 130, 134
House of Representatives, 51, 66, 125
household income, 29
housing, ix, 15, 31, 32, 93, 119
Housing and Urban Development, 95
housing benefit, ix, 31, 32
human, 96, 127
human resources, 96, 127

I

improvements, x, 52
in vitro, viii, 2, 9, 10
income, viii, xi, 1, 3, 4, 5, 7, 20, 22, 23, 24, 25, 26, 28, 29, 36, 89, 91, 117, 118, 119, 136
independence, 12
independent living, 99
Indians, 28
individuals, 22, 23, 38, 42, 57, 117, 120
infection, 12, 83, 85, 86, 88
infertility, viii, 2, 10
inflation, 44, 95
information technology, 93, 94, 136
infrastructure, 96, 127
injury(s), ix, 5, 6, 13, 15, 18, 25, 33, 34, 37, 39, 42, 52, 59, 91
insane, 35
insanity, 35
institutions, 28
insurance policy, 18, 46
integrated health care delivery system, vii, 1, 66
Internal Revenue Service, 136
intervention, ix, 52, 59
ionizing radiation, 20, 23, 117
Iraq, 8, 110
issues, x, 38, 52, 53, 57, 59, 67, 82, 86

J

jurisdiction, 129
justification, 125, 135

L

labeling, 125, 131, 134
layperson, 28
lead, 16
leadership, 59, 83
legislation, 106
life expectancy, 86
light, 27
loan guarantees, 91
loans, 37, 42, 119
logistics, 127

M

majority, 48, 91
management, 11, 12, 55, 59, 65, 68, 71, 72, 73, 74, 79, 80, 81, 83, 84, 88, 96, 121, 127, 128
Marine Corps, 33
mark up, 107
marriage, 45
Maryland, 28
materials, 75
matrix, 54
matter, 18, 55, 58
median, 119
Medicaid, vii, 2, 7, 23, 28, 46, 91, 117, 119

medical care, vii, viii, ix, xi, xii, 1, 2, 7, 10, 14, 19, 20, 28, 41, 42, 48, 60, 89, 90, 91, 93, 95, 97, 100, 105, 106, 107, 110, 119, 124, 125, 126, 127, 129, 130, 131, 132, 133
Medicare, vii, viii, 2, 7, 18, 19, 21, 22, 28, 46, 47, 48, 91, 97, 106, 119, 121
medication, viii, 2, 10, 17, 19, 20, 26, 98
medicine, 60
membership, 9, 39
mental health, 7, 9, 47, 110, 126, 129, 130, 135
methodology, 68
Miami, 67, 82, 83
military, vii, viii, ix, xi, 1, 2, 3, 4, 5, 6, 10, 12, 20, 22, 24, 25, 26, 27, 31, 32, 33, 34, 36, 37, 38, 44, 45, 49, 89, 91, 118, 119, 120, 122
minimum service requirements, vii, 1, 34
Missouri, 67, 82, 83
mucous membrane(s), 86
multiple sclerosis, 13

N

National Defense Authorization Act, 5, 119
national emergency, 39
National Institutes of Health, 97
NCA, xi, 89, 91
nurses, 56
nursing, viii, xii, 2, 13, 14, 15, 19, 28, 47, 99, 116, 124, 126, 127, 132, 133, 136
nursing care, viii, 2, 14, 47, 116
nursing home, xii, 13, 15, 19, 28, 99, 116, 124, 126, 127, 132, 133, 136

O

Obama, 7, 105
Obama Administration, 105
Obama, President Barack, 7
occupational therapy, 14
Office of Management and Budget, 106, 122, 123, 127, 135
officials, x, xi, xiii, 52, 53, 55, 56, 57, 59, 64, 65, 67, 68, 70, 72, 73, 74, 75, 76, 77, 78, 79, 81, 82, 83, 84, 86, 87, 124, 125, 126, 129, 131, 132, 133, 134, 137
OMB, 106, 122, 123, 127, 129
Operation Enduring Freedom, 119
Operation Iraqi Freedom, 119
operations, 4, 5, 26, 91, 96, 119, 120
oral health, 11
organ, 12, 47
outpatient, viii, ix, xi, xii, 2, 7, 9, 16, 17, 20, 47, 51, 59, 66, 89, 95, 96, 98, 124, 126, 127, 136
oversight, vii, xi, xiii, 42, 64, 65, 67, 68, 76, 77, 78, 79, 80, 81, 82, 83, 84, 86, 87, 95, 96, 121, 124, 125, 126, 129, 130, 134, 135

P

palliative, 9
participants, 48
pathology, 14
patient care, 55, 59
peer review, 53, 55, 56, 57, 60, 61
permit, 35, 136
Persian Gulf, 4, 36, 37
Persian Gulf War, 4, 36
pharmaceuticals, viii, 2
photosensitivity, 13
physical therapy, 14
physicians, ix, x, 52, 53, 57, 60
planned action, 81
policy, x, xiii, 52, 53, 54, 57, 58, 60, 61, 68, 71, 75, 84, 86, 124, 126, 137
population, 83, 85, 88, 136
preparation, 87, 127
prescription drugs, 9, 20, 47, 119, 126
President, xi, 7, 89, 91, 93, 96, 99, 100, 101, 102, 104, 105, 106, 107, 108, 109, 110, 111, 112, 114, 120, 128, 135, 136, 137
prevention, 110
prisoners, 3, 13, 17, 22, 24, 136
prisoners of war, 3, 13, 17, 22, 24, 136
private sector, 99

project, 127
prostheses, 47
prosthetic device, viii, 2
protection, 91, 96
PTSD, 109
public health, 96

Q

quality assurance, 60

R

radium, 20
recall, 65, 71, 72, 81
recognition, 42
recommendations, 58, 61, 64, 68, 80, 81, 84, 87, 124, 135
recovery, 97
Reform, xii, 3, 7, 26, 90, 92, 100, 104, 105, 107, 108, 111, 114, 120, 137
refresher training, x, 52
regulations, viii, 2, 10, 38, 49, 121
rehabilitation, 11, 12, 91, 99, 121
Rehabilitation Act, 121
rehabilitation program, 11, 12, 99
reimburse, viii, 2, 16, 18, 116
relevance, 67
reliability, 60
remediation, x, 52
repair, 120, 127
reprocessing, xi, 64, 65, 66, 67, 68, 69, 70, 71, 72, 73, 74, 75, 76, 77, 78, 79, 80, 81, 82, 83, 85, 86, 87
reproductive oncology, viii, 2, 10
requirements, vii, ix, xi, 1, 4, 10, 14, 26, 31, 32, 33, 34, 37, 41, 60, 64, 65, 66, 67, 68, 69, 71, 72, 74, 76, 77, 78, 79, 80, 81, 82, 83, 84, 86, 87, 91, 108
researchers, 97
reserves, 37
Residential, 15
resolution, 106, 107
resource allocation, 126
resources, 3, 4, 15, 28, 60, 108, 120, 127, 128, 132, 136, 137
response, x, 52, 60, 67, 68, 73, 75, 84, 87, 88, 129, 132, 135
restrictions, 61
retirement, 29
revenue, 95, 97
risk(s), ix, x, 52, 53, 54, 55, 60, 64, 65, 66, 67, 68, 72, 75, 76, 77, 78, 79, 80, 83, 84, 85, 86, 87
risk management, x, 53
root, 53, 54, 55, 56, 57, 60
rules, 45, 90, 106, 120

S

safety, x, xi, 52, 53, 54, 60, 64, 65, 66, 67, 69, 71, 72, 74, 75, 76, 77, 78, 79, 80, 82, 83, 85, 86, 87, 88
school, 28, 45
scope, 10, 58, 68, 84, 87
Secretary of Defense, ix, 32, 37, 38
security, 96
Senate, xii, 51, 66, 90, 100, 101, 102, 104, 105, 106, 109, 111, 112, 114, 115, 120, 122, 125, 126, 129, 130, 134
service provider, xi, 41, 89, 91
shortfall, 108
skin, 86
smoking, 17
Social Security, 22, 28, 29
social services, 14
social support, xi, 41, 89, 91
speech, 14
spending, 42, 105, 106, 107, 120, 129, 134
spinal cord, 15
stabilization, 18
staff members, 56, 73
staffing, 99
state(s), 4, 6, 14, 21, 39, 57, 60, 61, 85, 87, 91, 96, 97, 110, 116, 120, 127, 130, 132
statutory authority, 97
sterile, 86
stroke, 5, 6, 13

structure, xiii, 69, 95, 124, 126, 129, 130, 134, 135
subacute, 131
substance abuse, 9, 47, 120
suicide, 110
supervision, 15, 68, 84, 87
supervisor, 56, 61
support services, 15, 96
survivors, vii, viii, ix, 1, 7, 10, 41, 42
symptoms, 42, 121

T

target, 82
taxation, 118
TBI, 109
technical comments, 58, 81, 136
teeth, 11
telephone, 17, 27
temporary appointment, 59
testing, viii, 2, 13, 20, 23, 87, 117, 121
therapy, 98, 99, 120
time frame, 81
time periods, 36
tissue, 86
Title I, 106
Title II, 106
tooth, 11
toxic substances, 3
toxicity, 13
tracks, 57
trainees, 91
training, x, 5, 7, 12, 33, 39, 52, 55-58, 65, 71, 73, 74, 75, 79, 80, 81, 86, 87, 91, 96
training programs, 96
transparency, 126
transplant, 12
transportation, viii, 2, 16
trauma, viii, 2, 10, 11, 20, 120
traumatic brain injury, 13
Treasury, 121
treatment, viii, 2, 10-14, 16, 17, 18, 20, 23, 25, 26, 28, 70, 95, 117, 120, 136
triggers, 56

U

unit cost, 95, 128
United, v, vi, ix, 22, 28, 34, 45, 51, 63, 66, 86, 96, 123, 125
United States, v, vi, ix, 22, 28, 34, 45, 51, 63, 66, 86, 96, 123, 125
universities, 97
updating, 137

V

variables, 83, 85, 88
variations, 25
vascular system, 86
Veterans Health Administration (VHA), vii, ix, xi, 1, 2, 41, 51, 84, 89, 91, 92, 121, 124, 126
Vietnam, 22, 23, 27, 29, 36, 39, 42, 97, 117, 119, 123, 131
vision, viii, 2, 13
vocational rehabilitation, 12, 23, 91, 93, 94, 117, 118

W

wages, 29
walking, 27
war, 4, 7, 11, 22, 23, 28, 36, 38, 39, 42, 91, 110, 117
Washington, 25, 27, 28, 49, 61, 85, 86, 87, 88, 121, 122, 136
water, 73
weight loss, 17
workers, 120
workload, 97, 137
World War I, 3, 22, 36, 38
wrongdoing, 61

X

x-rays, 11, 19